THE FIGHT FOR MY LIFE

BOXING THROUGH CHEMO

To Beth,

Thank you for your work
+ commitment to making
Nashville a stronger community.

Kelly Motley

with love,

Kelly Motley

To loves of my life:

John,
Will and Alex

Prologue

DRESSING ROOM

There's a strange thing about being on the wrong side of an ambush and not having time to process things in an ordinary manner. The unsuspecting, the element of surprise from concealed positions, this is what ambushes are built on. Advancing before anyone really knows what's taking place. We watched, hoped and waited.

It was a total of twelve hours, a full day and another half-day, sitting with a calm anxiousness, my husband John and I together, in the oncologist's waiting room for what was to be my first round of chemo through my new port on October 25. In life you don't see things playing out like this. We had met with the doctor the day before, been given our script for the production; it was direct and simple. We knew our lines, the important sequences of the day, had memorized details and each moment of action, and we could regurgitate the new order composed of check-ins, long waits, standing up after hearing my name called by a lab tech, checking my blood count to ensure proper functioning of my kidneys and liver, then we'd go off to the infusion area where pre-meds are given 30 to 60 minutes prior to the chemo to reduce nausea and allergic reactions.

I had spent three months visualizing this very day, sketching out each detail. Today's appointment was scheduled at least a month before, yet now I had a bad feeling. None of what we anticipated occurred. Everything about the expected experience would be all wrong. Instead of getting the chemo treatment with its sinister side effects, it all felt harmless. The day of waiting was unremarkable, unexpectedly delightful, ending with John and I leaving the doctor's office to go on a late afternoon date, to vote in an early election at the Belle Meade City Hall, enjoy an early vegan dinner and work out together at the Y. What I didn't know was there was a scheming vested interest and methodical manipulation at play, that was part of an obnoxious 12-hour wait for chemo, that would test my pride and will. The best way to tire out an opponent is to apply pressure. Waiting became the pressure fighting technique to tire me out.

However, the new reality could not be denied, only delayed, and I returned for my first chemo treatment. After a half-day of waiting, a door flew open and a nurse called my name, announcing my new destination. It would be difficult to move. My legs would feel heavy as if in a nightmare, struggling to trudge forward. We wandered down a long corridor to a place where the new geography seemed far from home, but was only three miles away.

All this time I had tried so hard to devise my own story, and here is where I recognized it all as a delusion. It was now I realized what I lacked: a fundamental grasp of the disastrous situation. You don't have to be hit in the face to be taken to that dangerous place where you are tested emotionally, to tap your will and character. I paused to see for the first time what human beings had contrived: a large, free-standing rectangular room filled with rows of buttery leather recliners called clinical infusion chairs.

Each chair came with its own IV pole. I entered a precarious reality, a packed, big-box, institutionalized supercenter of chemo. A place where I saw no favoritism. On the face of it, I might have looked like a newcomer to an AA meeting or someone watching a parade with the mishmash of ordinary people from all walks of life. We'd all be ordinary, condemned to recline together in the same strange posture, our feet pointed in the same direction, arms dangling or stretched out, empty handed, all of us bruised in the same spot, grown old before our time, with maybe an unavailable future. Exposed slaves to the lasting damage, docile, crossing a shadow line, so full of tears and sadness—the elderly holding onto walkers, the too young, the expectant mothers, some close to dying and exhausted, some with full heads of hair, some with bald heads wearing hats, others with wigs, some calm, deflated bodies, some weeping, smiling, the destitute, the rich, the crippled, active, heavy and thin, all together for a common cause, while eating pizzas and candy, drinking cans of soda, reading books. Some were subdued, others making conversation with friends or family.

Each person when going home would stare into a mirror and say: "No this is not me, I can't recognize myself." I now was experiencing the October 8 message of the day I had read for years in my great-grandmother Opal's AA 1971 book: "God or a spirit of the universe drawing *all* the people, us all together, to get closer to him through our common difficulties, dangers, and sorrows." Or it was a shared enemy uniting us all.

There were people moving swiftly between those who were stuck to poles and tubes, living their lives in parallel. At first sight, everything that happened was designed around a steady stream of young African-American women briskly walking from behind a counter. The counter resembled a trendy chef's counter restaurant designed to create a relationship, a dialogue with its customers where we get a front row seat to see the hum of swamped cooks on the line, always on display, watching them prepare our meal. These young aides exposed their patients and, in a roundabout way, themselves, through the administration of dangerous, strong, toxic potions, while also wrapping them in folded perfect squares of white, heated blankets and passing around enormous baskets of candy. Oncologists walked down a spacious polished and shiny corridor, looking away in a different direction, where no one is dying, avoiding eye contact with the reclining crowd in the spacious room that represented the horrors of the battle, seeing us only in their designated private offices, away from the day's effects of the deadly drugs.

Holy shit was my feeling; this is what my universe was now reduced to. Everything I felt I knew was now distorted. I'd never seen this as my reality. I was joining this new mortal team where just about everyone looked frumpy, wearing sweatpants. I found the place of aborted dreams and swallowed up hopes unbearable, reeking of decay, and I hated *It* even more now—*It* being this cancer thing and the bad situation I couldn't get out of, the wickedness and poor timing intended to wound each person's life. I grasped the simple truth in this space: *We are all going to die and all be forgotten.* It was here that I saw the exact opposite of paradise.

I had an impulse to turn back and run fast but I shuffled my feet forward with a forced smile at times, not meeting anyone's eyes, as if no one here existed. I struggled to breathe easily and could not think. I was tough on myself for having taken time to purchase expensive clothes and Alexander Wang boots to empower myself—boots I saw as "jungle boots" to help me march through these twelve rounds of chemo. I'd had a naive notion that if I dressed well, I'd be mentally stronger and be treated with more respect, which might equate to fewer medical errors. Or maybe I didn't want to dress for the part; maybe I wanted to impress others or be perceived as someone important.

All of a sudden, I shrank, feeling careless in my planning, and I was thrown off balance. I reflected back on a simple sentence 20-something year-old Sena Agbeko, who had knowledge beyond most men and had trained to be the next world champion of boxing from Ghana, told me matter-of-factly and frequently: "If you fail to prepare, you prepare to fail." I strived to understand how my opponent would work, with the goal to keep my opponent in an uncomfortable place, to make opportunities to control the fight. Every day was about breaking down the forensics of the fight. Until now, I thought I devised a well thought out fight plan. Now I experienced hesitation: It's one thing to make a plan and it's another to actually execute it.

I had tried my best—eating clean, getting physically and mentally stronger, and surrounding myself with the best of trainers to make a difference. The night before my first infusion, I'd followed strict instructions to eat salmon, medicinal foods and other protein that my nutritionist Virginia said, "would serve as a buffer along with Nishime, shitake mushrooms, Kinpira composed of a Japanese sea vegetable called kombu, along with burdock root, lotus root and a long, oblong white radish called daikon along with a side of black mahogany rice to settle the stomach." She had told me, "Breast cancer is from doing too much for others and giving too much out. Learn to have downtime and de-stress and you are going to feel your body shifting." I worked on all these things. Somehow, I had overlooked details like selecting an accessible doctor willing to meet with me through the treatments and mentally preparing for the appalling near-nakedness of lying back in what felt like the ultimate open floor plan while taking chemical infusions meant to heal.

My world was getting ready to be turned upside down as I was caught cold. I had tried to be rational. No amount of mental preparation would have made me ready for this. Once I found my chair there would be an apparatus used to bring me down or as an agent of distraction when I thought things had finally fallen into place. It was a simple IV pole with its plastic tube that was attached to the vein near my heart through a soft catheter. Then there would be a calculated perpetual wait, us watching nurses go by, keeping us in suspense. We froze when we saw them coming. In a civilized world, women aren't supposed to make these kinds of decisions about their life while a crowd of nurses, a business office administrator with paperwork and pens insist on a much more sinister type of treatment dictated by an insurance company. The day and a half in the waiting room and this ambush felt engineered to suit the desires of a few. Everything was so arranged.

It was here I was pushed to the brink, where I felt threatened with defeat. I was dragged into a fight I wouldn't be prepared for. I might have experienced this thing called panic fighting. Now I knew what my coaches meant by the phrase *calculated chaos*.

***

Everything that happened, led me to where I am meant to be. Sometimes you have to go through very difficult things, tortuous times, to get to a better place in life. This is my story about getting into the boxing ring with discomfort and chaos. It's a story about how I thought I knew how to play the system. I thought I had all the answers. I had a vision of the kind of person I wanted to be. But I was blindsided by a devastating blow. And then I got knocked down hard by a series of pummeling jabs that forced me to rethink everything. I bound up my wounds the best I could.

Boxing became my remedy, to uphold and guide me to make the right decisions, something to turn to for a higher help. I needed healing and was told by a man with a shaved head, who I would one day resemble, that self-pity took energy and would be useless. I'd get trainers telling me "No" when I wanted to give up, when I was about to fall—telling me to keep moving forward, encouraging me to keep pushing, reminding me this was not permanent. It was grueling and exhausting. And just when I thought there wasn't an ounce of energy left to pick myself up … ding-ding-ding, the fight for life was on!

Smug in my vision that I was the one making the good and proper

choices, nothing seemed arbitrary. There was my own self-import-
ant ordering of the world built around my value of trust, attributes
I had acquired and avoided, decisions I'd made in assessing other
people—people I wanted to stand far from and people I admired
most—all to make me who I was. I collected the best and avoided
the worst in what I experienced from people growing up.

The certainty that I was right about most things, about how one
lives a good life, what I had been chasing this whole time—the
rules I had been taught and how I solved problems all started
to unravel. I craved external validation, an artificial euphoria of
feeling successful and building my sense of worth.

My boxing training became a lesson for me because I had learned
things too late in life. I collapsed in my own ignorance. I was
getting a life lesson that I wasn't finished yet. In some ways it felt
like a second chance, a last hope to get things right, to get set free
or to straighten out. I might have been summoned here to learn
what matters most. Other times, it felt like a cruel joke that these
universally accepted principles existed all along and I was just
now exposed to them.

In each chapter, I share what got me through breast cancer. This
is the beginning of my breast cancer story. It starts in a rather
uncommon place for a middle-aged, professional southern white
woman with a PR business, married for 25 years and a mother
of two sons. The story begins in a concrete block building, previously an industrial plant, vacated for fifteen years before it
became a boxing gym. Boxing is a test of will and skill. I'd need to

focus on my conditioning, become mentally tough and surround myself with trainers endowed with physical and mental assets beyond those of ordinary people, trainers who pushed me hard to be mentally, physically and spiritually fit.

The universe was kindly, quietly guiding and giving me the very best to equip myself as I was unknowingly getting ready for one of life's biggest duels, one that would test my courage and willingness to change. Looking back on it, my training would be a time of design and preparation.

It was a stroke of luck to discover boxing before cancer. I surprised myself. I somehow assembled a group of elite trainers, locked together with me, to hold me up and keep me balanced and my mind undisturbed. Everything in my training pointed toward this new fight—cancer. It would be that one boxing match that would be a demonstrated test of my courage, hope and intelligence. The training would teach me new tricks every step of the way and make powerful shifts in my thinking, while supplying me with extraordinary physical strength and power in a time of need. It was a delicate thing, God giving me the chance to reimagine myself through a sport of fighting with fists inside a squared circle. "Everything you need is in your hands," said my minister-lawyer friend Robin, referring to Moses' staff and the power of truth. God put cancer and boxing in my hands to help me start fresh.

Boxing not only gave me a life lesson, but it literally and figuratively saved my life. I had no idea about the commonality of boxing and cancer. The common denominator is a simple intention to survive—bound in a place of pain, cruel humiliation and awful pressure where the beating can be severe. Each boxing match is a psychological drama, one of a kind. I'd see how devastating the opponent could be, testing the outermost limits where anything can happen and things can feel hopeless. I would be half-naked at times, cut and bleeding, bruised, swollen, where there is no hiding, and oftentimes losing control. Looking back, boxing and cancer became metaphors for each other: with two principal characters—you and it—the circumstance becomes fiercely personal, involving vulnerability, despair and endless courage. There are unsettling punches that take you by surprise, that punish the mind, body and spirit. The unpredictability, the rounds, the determination of the body and the awareness of the seconds ticking down. Where death is plausible. I would need to fight to the end, as if I didn't want to die.

What I discovered was that sweating it out by working mitts during chemo seemed to detoxify my mind and body, giving me renewed energy and focus. The power of these activities gave me an edge to make it through.

I surrounded myself with the very best of coaches, good and caring people in my corner. Each day was about learning *how* to discipline my mind, and how the body and mind must work in harmony in the toughest of workouts or in the boxing ring. While I was working on being able to adapt my mind, I also was trying to understand my coaches' technical instructions and then condition my body to respond. My coaches helped me to become well-trained mentally and physically, to gather the *right* mental tools and heightened focus I needed to change my energy, and to create a plan for taking on what was to be one of my life's biggest tests.

I never took one second of my training for granted. My notebook and pen were flung out of my backpack at the end of each training session as I meticulously captured my coaches' word-for-word feedback and knowledge. Videos of my progress were made, reviewed in detail, and then shared with me by my coaches. While everything was relevant to making me physically stronger or better in the ring, each training experience also related to helping me manage clients, grow my business, and be a better version of myself.

There are very few things in my life I feel I've been remarkable at. But recovering and bouncing back from chemo was a definite victory, thanks to my boxing training leading up to the diagnosis and during treatment. My corner, the people I looked up to, told me I turned into a top fighter, landing a massive knockout win over cancer. Sena wrote to me: *You are a better version of yourself in boxing now—coming back better than you were before. You are better than you think.*

I didn't want to die nor did I want this diagnosis to mean a wasted year of my life. My strategy was about having the best possible good endgame, and that included having non-complicated surgeries with quick recoveries and minimal downtime.

But I would get knocked down hard.

Round One

ALEX'S WRESTLING SHOES

Years ago, when my youngest son Alex was in middle-school, I felt undone by his participation on a wrestling team. The sport of wrestling, the combat part, tormented me. All I had to do was to look down at Alex' black-and-white Adidas wrestling shoes to bring me anxiety and panic. These shoes represented a string of negative images, my beads of perspiration, my wincing thoughts and tense feelings of Alex's damage and me feeling frozen. There I was, grimacing at my son in these shoes while he was wearing a tight-fitting, second-hand thinning Lycra one-piece maroon singlet, with opponents putting him in choke holds and head-locks, seeing him execute and receive takedowns and cradles in tight battles, sometimes with his face being smashed into the mat, his body being bent and twisted, and fighting back. These shoes brought back memories of my stomach lurching while I was secretly hiding out in the women's bathroom, inside a stall, flooded with anxiety; or uncomfortably sitting in the metal stands and showing an artificial enthusiasm as I cheered for my son.

I felt diminished in giving kindergarten-like instructions to his tough-talking coach, a former star wrestler at West Point, telling him that my son Alex would not be cutting weight. He said "Yes, I understand," but he meant: *No, that won't be happening* and he put my growing son on a treadmill without water or meals. I felt coerced to understand and wrap my arms around this sport that never made Alex smile but seemed more of a strange obligation, a relentless, enduring grind. There were the disturbing morning-after breakfasts—our family sitting at the breakfast table, three sets of eyes darting away from Alex in disbelief between mouthfuls of French toast, my husband John, older son Will and I sitting with a quiet worry for what had happened the day before to Alex's smooth, fair skin—now all bruised black and blue, with rosy, scaly circular patches. It felt like I was failing to keep him safe, failing as a parent.

Alex's shoes were a reminder of me squinting to recognize him limping down a long, bricked-over hilltop from after-school wrestling practices, the sun going down behind him, all bent over, careful with each step like a broken-down old man. The smallest glance down at these shoes brought traces of shame, with me reflecting back on the unusual liberty I took to sip a big dose of Cosmopolitans in a 44-ounce martini glass before noon to make it through an all-day Saturday regional meet. I wished Alex would announce that he was quitting.

But then I attended an all-boys school wrestling team banquet, and I realized, heard and saw how he felt the sport was like surviving something powerful. That evening, middle school parents and wrestlers waited for what Alex was going to say next. I was shocked to see the eyeballs all looking up, the moms, dads and boys all synchronized. He built the case of how wrestling had transformed him and brought him to adulthood early. Speaking with the authority of an adult and an attentive storyteller, and possessing a quiet confidence, Alex delivered a "Life isn't easy, take responsibility for your decisions, there will be hard choices" message. I watched forks drop, phones were cast aside, and no one glanced down at a watch. Here was this little boy with yellow hair, wearing khakis and a hand-me-down plaid shirt, explaining to the crowd: "If there is something you don't want to do, or need to do, or fear it, the best way to deal with it is to attack it and not run from your problems." I saw him standing effortlessly at the podium and had a flashback to a constant warning from a discerning neighbor-friend who said to always keep a close eye on Alex. "He's too cute and someone is likely to steal him."

I heard this boy tell the crowd that night: "Wrestling changed me, made me look differently at tough obstacles and adversity; it makes me face my fears and pushes me to go places I might have not gone otherwise, or tried to avoid. It has taught me many life skills—the tough practices, and how you can push through things, the self-discipline and how you can push your mind and body beyond a capacity never imagined." Looking back, this speech from my child could have been directed at me, a pep talk before my denial around a cancer diagnosis.

What I learned was how the most inconceivable in life happens when you start to believe again. Things change: the harshest of negative associations around feeling fearful—things, people, situations you might feel you'll hate for eternity—are all temporary and can flip at any moment.

I felt a reset about the harm these shoes represented when I pulled them out of my own gym bag. I thought about being quickly transformed as I slid my toes and heels into these shoes, tied the laces, and my heart began to beat faster. There were other events, like me wearing these shoes, that were also unthinkable, particularly at the age of 50.

***

Before I started boxing, I felt a dull, hard resignation that I would forever be stuck. Not stumbling, or even stumbling forward— just stuck. I wrote in my journal at the time that I was *in a state of lack*. Feeling good about myself felt like a Herculean effort. My 1924 house, my career and 25+ years of marriage felt like a struggle, a frustration, a quiet desperation. Every rickety thing in our home was breaking, from the impossible-to-fix drips of old faucets and light fixtures that would go out and then never work again to a pile of cinder blocks used as a back step. This home, where I worked and lived, screamed *survival mode*.

I lacked the backbone and kept my defenses down. I felt a deep sense of powerlessness in my life.

The relationship with a major client at the time felt daunting—a bout that just went on and on, every day so unevenly matched, outweighing me. The first six months I was conscious of his cheers. Then everything turned to devalue, and then discard. Every day, I felt knocked down by a blow I didn't see coming. All the while I was making my CEO client wildly rich and famous in his industry, but the boos seemed to be getting louder. My voice constricted on our calls as though I was being punched in my throat. I felt like I had no recourse. A full day of writing and practicing my talking points to help control the outcome of a meeting was a desperate attempt; I'd be cut off in a just a few minutes, and my carefully constructed plan would look like improvisation, thrown haphazardly together. My emotions swung from anxiety and feeling shut down, to fear of being shamed, and then anger. While I was getting a constant beat of media coverage for this client, I was stressed about our contract. No matter how hard I tried, I couldn't manage to get a needed signature.

One day things inside me broke. To pull myself back from the brink, I felt compelled to go punch something *that very day*. At the end of that work day, I backed my car out of a pea gravel driveway and drove down the road a few miles to a popular franchise boxing-inspired or box-exercise gym, where I pounded a bag, throwing hard, flailing, angry punches in a group class. I could have been mistaken for someone with Tourette syndrome, uncontrollably blurting out a string of words like "motherfucker." I saw my client's face right there on the bag. Pounding the bag, sweating, breathless with anger, raw aggression and rage seemed easy for me, so natural.

I was certain, given my emotional predicament, I'd be good at this boxing thing. I did not realize that in boxing, just like in life, the angrier you are, the more careless you become, the more you introduce risks, the more you negatively impact your breathing, form, and desired outcome. I purchased what was presented as a great deal, a membership along with *their* very best boxing gloves, oversized and intended for a man with hulking hands, vinyl with a Velcro strap.

The spirited instructors weren't real boxers but gifted athletes, former Division 1 college football players, state championship wrestlers and a professional ballerina. My younger son Alex and I would go together to the boxercise gym classes where we were caught by surprise at times, celebrated as though we were an extraordinary mother-son team. Walking through the front door with our bags filled with wraps and gloves, I felt reinvented when I'd see an instructor, wearing a microphone headset, approach us during his ongoing class to hold us up, announcing to everyone, "Look, here they are, here's two of our favorite clients." Alex at 13 was the youngest member, and I might have been the oldest at 50—together we became special.

I thought the classes would somehow save me. Exasperated with the conflict at work, there were days I took back-to-back classes. I stood there completely illiterate to the art of boxing, never moving my feet or hips, nor pivoting, not understanding how to be snappy or bend at my knees to execute a crisp roll, not once moving my head or stepping. Always having my guard down, I threw nothing but static, wild punches to a basic choreographed routine of jab, bob, weave and hook.

While punching a bag later in the day, I appealed to a higher power in the mornings. I combined these boxing-inspired work-outs with prayer and meditation. Before starting work, I sat in an upright position, cross-legged on the floor holding a palm-sized book designed for people "who drink, even when they don't want to, when they say they won't, but do." It was part of my haphazard approach to becoming a better version of myself. Using alcohol as a distraction to cope with the angst of life wasn't my dilemma. But I felt the same brokenness of a blind drunk, knowing that things had run amok, giving up on myself, battered, down on my luck, unable to find my desire. I thought it was a good time for me to surrender my self-will, get out of my own way, and turn my life over to a higher power using this 12-step AA thought-for-the-day meditation and prayer book. I was planning to do it the right way, to use this book to redesign my new life, unlike the book's original owner, Opal.

Opal was once exceptional, like all the other women in my mother's family—independent, tough, headstrong, an indestructible force. At the most inopportune moment at the end of WWII, while most American women were making beds, cooking meals and farming, Opal at age 40 reinvented herself in the charred ruins of the war-torn country of Japan. I never knew Opal as the polished, finely dressed piano playing woman from her photographs and eloquent letters, but as old, physically and mentally devastated from alcoholism.

I knew my courage was shrinking. I needed to change my direction, where I was retreating, by tapping into her spirit through this book, to show myself that nothing was impossible. I now felt bound to Opal and her demons—not because of a mutual love for alcohol, but because of our joint feelings of being in a blind alley. I thought I would make things right for both of us by meditating with her book.

And just when I thought I could keep my composure at work by meditating with a 12-step program, appealing to a higher power in the mornings and punching a bag later in the day, another obstacle to my sanity emerged.

Alex's interest in boxing spread to Mixed Martial Arts (MMA). He begged me to sign him up for a class at a popular tough-guy MMA school on the east side of Nashville, where the men assert their dominance by driving big trucks and look virtually identical with high levels of testosterone, heads held higher with dominance. It was here in this MMA gym I thought I might have walked into an organized underground fight club as I was watching Alex's first class. At his second class, I dropped him off in the parking lot, having arranged for my older son Will to pick him up. After the class, Alex opened Will's passenger car door with a crimson, friction-burned neck. He'd been choked out by the instructor in only his second class, Alex tapping the mat to end the match ("tapping out" is a quick way of saying I quit), then blacking out.

I was horrified and imagined the travesty of the situation, seeing this as a sadistic sport—Alex fighting to take a breath and his pain and physical suffering, with an adult man possibly putting his weight on his neck. I saw the bruises on his neck and in my mother's brain I was charged for my own carelessness. He and I sat quietly together on our sofa and he calmly spoke with no blame, sharing the details of his experience; what had transpired, the sensation of strangulation and blacking out.

I studied my son and thought back to that one award banquet

that would neatly summarize his reaction and show how my own doubts lead me astray. John and I had sat side-by-side, sweating for hours in a hot school gymnasium, our legs cramped from the confined space, confident of only one thing: all three of us had been mistakenly invited. Near the end of the program, with every lackluster academic award already handed out, I'd given up and was grabbing my purse and leaning forward to spring up, when I heard Alex's name called. It was a big deal award, with status in his school. I watched him walk to a podium to be recognized as the child who best represents a combination of kindness, compassion, modesty and forgiveness.

Listening to him talk about what and how the blackout happened, I also identified. I remembered as a 19-year-old college student I too had experienced this sensation of no longer being able to breathe, unable to physically fight for my life, pretty confident I was on the edge of being a victim of homicide—imagining what was happening as if I were across the room, people sitting down to read about my death in the news the next day, praying to God for intercession, pleading to even my dead father for help—when miraculously my ex-boyfriend released the force and pressure around my neck. I knew from my experience how such a person strangles to show he *can* kill, controlling victims with fear and intimidation. But *this* was about my 13-year-old son being choked in front of a group of non-interceding adult men, watching in this wide-open space.

I could only dream of what I wanted to do. I felt helpless and pondered all the details for several days, terrified to walk into the MMA school to face the instructor. All I could think to do felt wimpy. Summoning my courage, I called the owner of the MMA gym from a safe distance across town, on the other side of the Cumberland River, sitting at my dining room table. I kept myself calm as I confronted him with the details, just as if I was representing a client. I was scared to do this one small act for my son. What I recall is being shocked that he didn't twist the story but already knew what had happened. He unapologetically acknowledged with an audible shrug, "Yes." This call seemed to be squandering his time. I raised the subject of a refund. His response felt unremarkable, a loose end and insufficient.

I had managed PR for my clients as if I was my own authority, using techniques I had mastered a long time ago to get what I wanted in a simple conversation. But here, I surrendered, just shrank away and let it go. I felt incomplete; it wasn't enough. I was lost in understanding how to navigate my words. I fixated on this talk as being that one time in my life I wish I could have tried harder. Having this happen to my son was just another hint to expect nothing more than to keep putting up with everything.

I pondered all the details for several days as the MMA school burrowed inside me, me frightened to get too close to the instructor. I confided in the kind, muscly trainer-manager who worked the front desk of the boxing-inspired gym (the guy who sold me my membership and gigantic gloves). I gasped as this man shared common details of how he personally could relate to Alex's story at this MMA school. The manager was a former nationally ranked wrestler, and had been a Division 1 varsity college football player once looked at by the NFL, with a black belt in karate. He deliberately grabbed a yellow sticky-note pad from the counter and jotted down a phone number and the name "Richard Goodloe." He passed the sticky note to me without any explanation.

After a while, I began to feel that the man Richard on the yellow sticky note was a mythical figure or fiction, and I'd been set up to fail. The MMA chokehold and this Richard not returning my calls both felt like my own handbook in failure. The memorization of his phone number, the unreturned calls—more examples in my life of trying hard when my best wasn't good enough—defeated me. When Alex asked for a final update, I rolled my shoulders, hung my head and simply acknowledged in an exaggerated, overly pronounced fashion, "I ... tried ... my ... best," and I just gave up.

But unexpectedly one evening in the late summer, I found myself walking around in my front yard, talking on the phone with the elusive Richard. I listened to myself repeatedly saying "uh-huh" while getting a friendly tutorial around the principles of a "nothing is set in stone" form of martial arts called Jeet Kune Do, wondering if I was hearing him correctly when he talked about a few degrees of separation from Bruce Lee, a name I hadn't heard since the '70s. He was stressing that his lessons would most likely run longer than an hour. It all sounded good to me.

A few days later, my body felt heavy sitting on the portable heavy-duty aluminum and steel bleachers inside a dusty warehouse converted to a boxing gym. I noticed Richard watched every-one and everything with dedicated attention, with great inter-est. His instructions were cool, simple and neutral. Alternately humorous with critical examination, this man could have been a contemplative monk, or conceivably one of the most dangerous unarmed killers, ready to handle any combat situation with fists, a pen, knife or gun.

I sat quietly and at first, I didn't know what it was I was seeing. In an instant, the unexpected happened for me, a bending of space and time, and I saw an opportunity to reset myself. Like a fire in the sky, this Bruce Lee martial arts thing drew me in, telling me my fear was holding me back, bleeding into everything. *It was time to get life back on track.*

Alex was barefoot, wearing black hand wraps and boxing gloves. I watched him exploring what seemed the ultimate in human potential, maybe unlocking what I'd heard of "the third eye," in what looked like a street fight with hand-to-hand combat. He was instructed to land both explosive and snappy kicks, designed to go through an opponent rather than just kick the target— sometimes generated from the knee, other times from rotating the hip, leaning back and temporarily shifting his weight, with a focus on using his shin bone. I felt like an intruder, watching Alex going into a meditative flow with showy mitts. This Richard orchestrated fluid, telegraphed punches and kicks, twisting to the side at different angles. The combinations would be for speed and impact, incorporating both offensive and defensive move-ment to catch jabs and crosses, with Alex ducking punches while bending at the waist. There was a perfect distance between the two, with Richard absorbing the force of a punch or kick. Both of them made the experience look easy. The kicks I saw my son land were designed to impact the opponent's stability, directed at the knees, thighs, or midsection.

It all felt like a message. This experience was about thinking on your feet, taking a risk by confronting a difficult situation, trusting your gut. I saw something here I wanted: that thrill of pushing the envelope, of my center of gravity, by moving within and beyond my base of support without toppling over. After the lesson, I worked hard to express a toned-down, mild interest in what Alex was learning. Richard responded with a simple, "Well, c'mon then."

This was my turning point. Everything seemed too hard before this. Asking for something I wanted never felt this easy. But I worried for Richard that he might later feel remorse in his decision. Tangled up with so much frustration, I thought I could be his most complicated client.

On Saturdays, I stood side-by-side with my 13-year-old getting back-pocket life information, not available to everyone, based on a freedom of movement street-style combat fighting that comprised a see-move-feel ideology: realize there is no fixed way, know yourself, look at people without judgment, react to force with gentleness and, if you need to overcome it, use the shortest distance. Be open-minded, fluid, efficient, use your strongest weapon, and find the softest target. All this strangeness drew me in, rescued me.

We were standing in front of a man who was not a theory fighter. His steadiness, mild manner, unobtrusiveness, and sensitivity might be misleading. He did things that are essential to survival. He pointed out, without having to say the words, how the opponent the whole time was me. I heard things like: "Start thinking about what slows you down and stops you. Let the muscles do what they are supposed to do. Identify whatever you see in your head that is controlling and slowing you down." Then when he said I was "just tapping, not punching or kicking through," it all made sense. I understood how I was just going through the motions.

I was astonished to understand how power comes from being relaxed and comfortable. I had thought being successful was about intensity and taking everything seriously. I held my hands tight, arms locked in position, fixed, airtight, holding my breath, gasping at times as if underwater. Training frequently stopped. I'd be given a slow purposeful, curious look, followed by a question no one in my life had ever asked me. In a neutral tone, he'd ask me: "Are you breathing?" My look showed I was perplexed, later confirming I was neither breathing out nor in, but instead holding my breath. Everything was about trying too hard. I experienced for the first time how the simplest moves work the best, how being efficient conserves energy.

He strung together two words built around a space that is more than just a place we live in: *Go home*—a phrase built around the concepts of never going willingly, fighting to the death, and making sure the opponent doesn't get several tries. I heard this couple of words enough to make me wonder at which point should I turn to two other words: why bother. I had stopped valuing myself and just plain fighting for myself now felt strange.

He talked relentlessly about the body constantly negotiating between being relaxed and being in position, saying things like: "You have to train like you are in a real fight—train in uncomfortable situations; train with your tools in your hands. Start to see the things around you as weapons." In this space, being put in uncomfortable situations toughened me up. I started to learn how much in life I could control. Pushing myself beyond my mental limits forced me to find new ways to hold onto to a sense of calm, to make adjustments, no longer thrashing.

I agreed to being placed in and getting out of what would be the worst-case scenarios, where you automatically think *My time is up*, and your last words are *Oh, shit*. To be face down on the floor with a bigger and stronger someone on my back, being on the ground with this person standing over me, attacking from behind, or to be stalked and cornered with this imposing man moving towards me. Receiving explicit instructions for catching an opponent off-guard, throwing a person off balance and finding the quickest route for getting up off the floor or out of the corner brought new confidence, a strengthened fortitude, a change in my determination.

Watching Richard demonstrate a "Tactical Get Up" reminded me of a dynamic and daring contemporary dance move, with different rhythms and a multi-level movement in different spaces. He moved up and over and off the ground, safe and sound, before I knew it. He started on his back, palms on the floor, with his left knee well bent and foot planted on the ground, and straightened the other leg out. His right arm extended above the head in a swim-like motion, he pushed his hips up in the air with a smack, and then with his right leg extending straight off the ground, his foot kicked, aiming at an imaginary attacker's knee cap or right below. I wanted to own this choreography as my story, showing the ugly, unsettling aspects of life as well as the beautiful.

The first time in the ring, I was in one corner, Alex in another. Richard, the most physically imposing man I'd ever met in my life, was coming at me. I froze and put my hands over my eyes saying, "I'm scared out of my mind." The steps to get out of this desperate situation were carefully explained, and I later found myself flipping his 220-pound body over my head and back—leaving him on his back on the canvas floor.

I learned how the simplest of motions could feel like a hush to my body. With Alex standing alongside me at the end of an old clothesline, slightly touching the line at our shoulders, we moved back and forth laterally, weaving, bobbing and rolling under it. Initially, doing this one simple movement seemed to me pointless, irritating and boring. But working on this thing called slip drills started feeling like the simple, quick, back-and-forth calming movement of a rocking chair or the lulling sensation of looking up at the clouds. Mentally, making the simple adjustment to each side let me know I would no longer be a target.

My thinking changed around how I viewed common, conspicuous body parts that I was previously blind to, never really valued, such as my sharp-boned elbows and shins and soft tissue spots. I could see my hips that moved freely and my thighs and calves strong from years of dance. Now I was lured by the magnificence of elbows, not just for poking, but as powerful, sword-like weapons cutting through the air, much more effective than punching with fists in a moment's danger. The impact, the efficient movement of striking with my elbows, felt naturally fun. Richard stood in front of us to demonstrate how to efficiently make any man crack. He brought his fingers to a small vulnerable spot on his chest below his collar bone, a few inches from his armpit, for pressing and driving to most efficiently inflict pain.

Every week was about how to orient myself around specific steps to stay alert, to pay attention to my surroundings by practicing this new concept of situational awareness. I'd be given movies to watch for homework assignments. I became acquainted with the importance of avoiding confrontation and dangerous situations by learning to leave, plus ways to de-escalate. Form might not be relevant if attacked. It's not about getting in a correct boxing stance, as there are no rules or etiquette. There would be an unhesitating need to identify vulnerable soft-tissue spots and to seek and grab objects that could become weapons of opportunity (pens, the heel of a shoe, scissors, keys, stick, dirt, fingernails). In stunning a possible attacker, I worked to overcome the awkwardness of bringing attention to myself with a loud low-pitched scream to take action.

I used these principles to think about new ways to intercept negative client communications, to protect my business, to relax to perform well, and to always be able to recall the importance of breath. I started to make small moves, no longer locked up with indecisiveness. I made shifts, and I didn't care if they were awkward, clumsy steps. I just began to move and make changes.

I started these movements on calls with my difficult client. I had been leaving myself open to be taken advantage of and letting others have my power. Not being defensively responsible showed up in my boxing, and it showed up in my life. Before and during client conference calls, as a visual to be defensively responsible, I routinely got in my boxer's stance and threw what Richard taught me: simple, fluid relaxed jabs and crosses with slips, all while focusing on being solidly grounded with the earth.

After a few months of lessons, I struggled with memorizing combinations, a hybrid of showy kicking, punching, grappling and trapping techniques that looked good on camera but would also hold up in a street fight. Getting positive feedback from Richard on anything started to feel as if I was failing. I had an inexplicable compulsion for perfect boxing form and technique to show both Alex and Richard. To keep up, I'd need to deviate. Most people might consider it utterly insane. But for me to practice this form of martial arts, I needed to better understand boxing fundamentals, to gain a new certainty and confidence. To this end, I'd meet a man known by a nickname in the boxing world as a quiet killer.

Round Two

MERRY STREET GYM

This sport of boxing would lead me to a dead end, Merry Street. At first, I really didn't know where I was headed in the early morning mist, not understanding the neighborhood at all. Getting out of the coziness of my car, I thought my new boxing trainer was just being overly polite by greeting me with a slight bow and saying in the Queen's English, "Good morning and welcome" when meeting me outside the gym's door most mornings.

It was said there had been more crimes than white people on Merry Street. In the '80s and '90s, it had been a really bad drug territory. Dealers set up shop at the top of the hill, where a "serving" of crack was offered like a fast and efficient quick-service drive-through. On a street without stoplights, there were tales of car-jackings right in front of the gym. It's the type of community where, regardless of your color, you need to identify, understand and respect who is in charge; otherwise, you might get caught *slipping*, meaning hit in the head. The neighborhood was dramatically framed as a place that takes its toll. There would be some people not lucky enough to make it out. People would reroute around the street, as if there was an imaginary boundary, a travel advisory had been issued, or it was a combat zone.

When we were first getting ready to move to Nashville, our old Nashville white team of realtors raised their eyebrows and explained in a southern drawl that homes on the other side of

Charlotte Pike were sketchy, shabby, and broken into. No matter the warnings, this is where I was headed that first morning to meet a man professionally known as the African Assassin, Sena Agbeko. It was time for me to be really honest with myself, stop running away from life and start facing things as they are. I would be boxing in the 'hood. With unease at first, I crossed over Charlotte Avenue and bumpy train tracks into a Nashville neighborhood where most of the time I was the only white spot around. But for me, it was here that everything loosened. It got to the point where I wanted to be there all the time.

What I experienced three mornings a week was this thing called happiness. In my earlier work of promoting a global well-being index, I was directed away from ever using the word "happiness." A group of scientists insisted it was shallow and I *was dinged* if I ever landed one media story with the forbidden word "happy." But I began to wake up with a wide smile, similar to my fourth-grade school photo, confident, with a clear sense of purpose. I sprang out of bed, pulling my car onto a wide boulevard known in the city for its patriotism, privilege and a fraternity of the well-connected. On my way over to Merry Street, I was straightaway certain that I was the luckiest woman in the world.

The life I had led until this moment had not prepared me for the extraordinary phenomena I'd experience on Merry Street. What I saw as initially strange, foreign, or novel soon became an everyday routine. The drive into the neighborhood caused me to loosen, get untwisted, step away from the continuing humdrum: I was no longer troubled, no longer wanted approval, was not answerable, no longer moving aimlessly, and I'd let go of people's expectations and the need to impose my sense of order on the world. On my seven-minute commute, I slowed down to respect an area with its own mysterious rhythm. It was on this tangle of back streets that I landed where my soul needed to be.

At the top of the hill on Merry Street, I passed what would have been, in a long-ago era, a premier neighborhood grocery store, painted the color of enlightenment and optimism—a bright yellow. The vibrant color was faded, the building still standing but decaying. It had an energetic, bustling feel and remained a busy neighborhood gathering spot. The design and materials matched the church I just passed, built with the exact same cinderblock design and stair-stepped wall. Resha's Grocery resembled the outside of an old Western saloon with hitching posts for tying up a horse. At one time there would have been a jar of sugar cookies on the counter for kids, hardwood floors, and customers would have run monthly tabs. There might have been games going on at the back of the store. There was a boarded-up glass window where in the past a butcher handed out orders of freshly cut deli meat. I saw people pull up, get their basics and lottery tickets, and move on. By mid-morning most days, there was a group of men watching everything that passed, standing inside a fenced-in front yard that connected to the market's parking lot, hanging out as they whistled and called, "Hey, baby girl." I watched people come in and go out of a dense forested thicket behind Resha's and wondered what was going on. A man with his front teeth in gold went in to buy individual cigarettes for a $1 from a man born in a different country. I saw all the broken bottles around the building and thought it needed a good cleaning and some flowers planted.

I turned right, down a deserted dead-end street that concluded at railroad tracks. Dogs ran loose. I slowly navigated my car between a parked, rusty old RV and a medical supply delivery truck perfectly aligned on either side of the street. I shimmied the car around at the bottom of the hill, the end of the street with a tangle of viney trees and rubble, to park it facing Resha's. At the bottom of this hill, I was reminded of what would become my own private and new secret view of Nashville's skyline.

In this parking spot across from the gym, I faced a void next to me, and I was given a subtle hint that there was once a grand home, built with close attention and great expense. I had heard stories about the family home turned crack house that had been demolished by the city. Everything had been erased, leaving nothing behind but the five-foot brick columns and four brick steps built back when people first made a statement around curb appeal. Now it looked like a new urban countryside, a desolate field, lush greenery. For me, it had a haunted feel, the absence of this home, the lost history and forgotten memories. Few homes were spared on Merry Street, mostly dominated by vacant lots.

In a real-life version, I also was bearing witness to a visual pattern—the disquieting plight of a neighborhood—a rigorous sweeping away of African-American churches, daycare centers and homes—a steady shrinking of a community and its final surrender. Each day another building was flattened and I recognized the demolition plot, an infiltration and carefully constructed operation to sabotage the smallest to the biggest of places and replace them with a prosperous white sector for living, working and shopping. There would be nothing left to remember. This seemed like part of a business deal, the tossing away of lives and homes like they never existed.

As I stepped out of the car and closed the door, my eyes and ears adjusted to this new place, looking at life around me with fascination. I pivoted my mindset, loosened the grip of what defines me like a snake shedding its skin. I greeted and talked to the same pale white man with a crumpled face of deep wrinkles and a permanent limp coming up the hill from the train tracks that cut across the bottom of the wooded street. Anywhere else, I would have looked away, maybe seen him as threatening, and would have done my best to avoid him. But here I'd say good morning and lock eyes with him. I studied his face to conceptualize his age. He was either my age and had a rough life or he could have been 30 years older and served in Vietnam. He walked in the early mornings as if he'd turned a chapter in his life, getting up to face a new day. I wondered about his story. I paid attention as I stepped over a thin crack in the street that stretches from the bottom of the hill all the way to the top.

I walked through an industrial 12-foot chain link fence that once protected a commercial two-story white cinderblock building, previously an industrial chemical plant, that had been vacant for fifteen years before. It was a boxing gym. I got inspiration from the entryway—a poster with Muhammad Ali's image and quote:

"I hated every minute of training, but I said, don't quit, suffer now and live the rest of your life as a champion." Alone and isolated on this dead-end street most mornings, I worked in complete trust with a professional super middleweight champion, knowing he could—not that he would—crush me with just his pinky.

There was the usual equipment you might find in a traditional boxing gym, along with an entire wall lined with mirrors where you could check in with your self-worth and form, no matter where you were standing. This place was not gritty, just raw with a methodological order and layout purposely designed around the science of the sport. Just like practicing good science, this gym would follow certain rules and guidelines. The logic here was to hone skills—balance, reflexes, coordination, tactical planning, analyzing the opponent and training the body to respond. An opened garage door in the back room brought in fresh air and a hilltop view of Nashville's spreading skyline. The visuals on the walls encouraged good reading habits, and there was a whiteboard for taking notes. Amateur and pro fighters would leave this gym for the prestige of training somewhere else with a big reputation in a faraway city, only to come back and realize how good they had it here.

For me, this Merry Street gym and this extremely masculine sport became an open window to escape a box of space and time, emptying my mind of limitations. There was no judgment in this place. No grades. I just got to be better at everything here. I learned that my body and mind must work in harmony both in the boxing ring and when transcending an obstacle in life.

It's where I was trained to run into unexpected punches, a place where I either defensively blocked them or slipped past by moving my head and torso to one side.

Round Three

THE AFRICAN ASSASSIN

There was a serendipitous chain of events that led me to end up training in the ring with Sena in the Merry Street gym. Strangely enough, it started with a casual conversation at my son Alex's Saturday afternoon baseball game with a blonde woman who worked at a law firm and carried herself with unapproachable authority. She was a boxer and married to a boxing coach. I explained I'd had a bad experience with an instructor at the boxercise gym and needed to learn boxing for my Jeet Kune Do. She recommended I train with Sena. But the notion seemed absurd. I could barely follow the scripts at the boxercise gym.

A few months later, I reached out to a USA 2012 winning Olympic boxing coach, author and Ph.D., Christy Halbert, who founded and led the nonprofit boxing gym on Merry Street. She too proposed I train with this boxer named Sena. My decision was fraught with hemming and hawing. But I was falling behind in my Jeet Kune Do training and needed a knowledge of boxing. I clung to Jeet Kune Do sessions as if my life depended on them. Something about this martial art felt like I was believing in myself again, getting divine assistance, my soul was feeling less weak and asleep. I was fearless in hopes of winning back my happiness, and working with Sena set off part of a grand design.

So, I began to see Sena three days a week. Most mornings, it was just the two of us training alone in this gym.

***

It's a rare morning. Today I get to try and punch a prizefighter, and he's 21 and 1 in his professional career. Sena Agbeko is known professionally as the African Assassin, the super middleweight professional boxer and 26-year-old from Ghana. I see Sena fitted in black leather headgear buckled under his chin, a mouthpiece and groin protector. In a fight, all the world knows Sena would always be the better opponent. At first glance, men look away and question whether they are sufficient. Women draw a discernable gasp. When I showed a picture of Sena to a friend, her immediate reaction was, "He looks fake." His muscles are like ironclad steel. His skin stretches *only* on top of muscles, with a single-digit percentage of body fat. His biceps, triceps, and deltoid region are chiseled and sculpted. He's 6-foot-1. The color of his skin is inherited from his kin in Accra, Ghana. He has a beautiful smile that shows grace and style. You see him and think there is no greater beauty than being born Black. His hair is closely trimmed by his ears with braids on top, pulled together into a spray of hair on his head. He has a square jaw, broad forehead, and high cheekbones.

The first few times I trained with Sena made me question myself. I was overcome by an irresistible impulse to run out without a backward glance. In the ring, I might have a nervous twitch, panic-stricken moments feeling foreign to this world I had landed in, unsure of the newness of what I was doing and who was training me. I recognized every second that I was violating my girlfriend Sarah's recommendation, a guided fundamental rule that

I'd held onto for 30 years: *Don't ever find yourself in a room with any man where a door can be closed and locked.* To compensate, I just closed my eyes at times, squinted, or my face might have twitched in spasm, expressions that said I just smelled something bad or was physically uncomfortable. But the goal was to end up with a neutral gaze. I heard Sena say calmly, "Relax the face." At times, when nothing made sense to me, I thought, *I can't believe I'm doing this*, then reminded myself why I was here.

If it's possible, he appears even more audacious in sparring equipment. I learn that our goal is for him to evade or "pass my punches" without retaliation. It's in this space where I'm forced to think about what it is to be human, to share a story where anything can happen. The common denominators are capability, the powers we possess, and being exposed. Here I live without the risk of ever getting hit.

I feel like I'm an imposter or I'm having an out-of-body experience. I'm being told in a distinctive Ghanaian pronunciation, "Quickly, let's get in the ring." Hastily climbing up onto a square raised platform, I bend down to step headfirst under the second white rope, threading my torso and legs into an empty ring that forms the boundaries of the competition area. The ring measures 16x16 inside the ropes, and I look down to see tiny crimson stains on the soft royal blue canvas mat. I tilt my head up to see what was becoming a familiar patriotic symbol of blood, wealth and freedom hanging from a ceiling of open-faced insulation— the proud flag of Ghana with a tricolor of red, gold, and green horizontal stripes, plus Marcus Garvey's inspired black pointed star in the center, representing the Pan African movement, freedom, and denouncing colonialism as a legacy of slavery and acts of indignity. In my mind, the flag's storyline would forever be linked to Sena's identity, this boxing character who incorporates these colors and star symbol into his boxing uniform for strength, power and presenting a greater narrative.

It's taken a while for me to feel like I deserve to be in a boxing ring. In retrospect, it was at first a chilling moment, feeling clumsy and unworthy. Now it's this space that gives me a psychological rush, feeling possessed of certain power and more qualified to do anything. Everything I see is in a brighter and sharper focus. Being in the ring activates a personal beat to the rhythm of my own core, a self-communion where the body, mind and soul unite. I see with different eyes, think with a different mind, and when I move it's more lucid and time feels slower than normal. Moving in circles in this space, my inside and outside all go together. Drawing my fists up by my chin here, I step with a focus on balance, keeping centered, never leaning too far forward or back. I gain confidence and footing in my own experience and story. It's my willingness to move in a circle here that will get me ready for what is coming: my suffering. I start to understand the need to put myself in an uncomfortable space and to train in that space. If I never do it this way, it will never come or I'll just go half-way, always with a hesitation. I work to stay in the centermost of the ring.

I warm up by shuffling around to the left perimeter of the ring with only a focus on well-controlled footwork and balance. Even with my dance background, I'm off most days in keeping my feet equally balanced as I move, staying in my boxer's stance while pushing off with my right foot when moving forward, and pushing off with my left foot when moving backward, pivoting when I get close to a corner, mindful to keep my feet continuously at an equal distance. I'm told to relax my face, keep my torso like a boat on the water, while my feet are moving in a smooth rhythm as though I'm jumping rope. With my hands in wraps and gloves, balled up by my tucked chin, throwing random jabs, I change direction. I throw my first signature punch combo: a double lead jab, cross, left hook, right hook, left undercut, right undercut, left hook, right hook. Then a double lead jab, slip to the left, slip to the right, right hook, left hook, right hook, left trigger, right hook, left hook, right cross, right trigger, right uppercut, left hook, right uppercut. I'm reminded to let my legs and feet drive the punches, rotate the hips more and get a greater extension with my jabs and crosses.

The bell rings, signaling the start of a three-minute round and turning my mind to immediate categorization: It's either *Go Time* or that's enough. There's a tap of gloves, like a handshake or salute, acknowledging that things are starting. We stand facing each other with our left arms slightly extended in front, right arms closer and crossing the chest.

It's a strange thing having a man (who blamed his only record loss at the time to overtraining by running 13 miles a day) moving toward you in a boxing ring. I initiate and try to set the tone. Staying relaxed while putting together rhythmic combinations for attack and defense, I visualize myself as a certain fighter, baiting, moving laterally, shifting, retreating, bobbing my head, making quick step-offs at a rapid pace, trying not to be predictable. Seeing an opening, I try to throw him off balance with a simple pause, jab, cross (pause) cross. I'm reminded again of "the principles of relaxation while being explosive, the power of breathing, to be snappy, think clearly and to make adjustments."

He shifts his body just a few inches and places himself out of range of every punch coming. I can't lay a glove on him, nor can I get within punching range. His shadow crosses over me like a phantom. I see a big grin through his mouthpiece. No matter which way I step, his presence feels like a conjoined dark shadow that I can't shake.

Sena keeps a watchful, neutral gaze. I'm keeping a good distance but start to question whether this is the appropriate range. I feel engaged in an unwanted, outsmarted, effortless chasing. It's quite possible that he is meditating or asleep with his simple inflow and outflow of breath. I'm wondering if he recognizes how his steady, quiet presence with skilled mirroring of movements becomes an awful, terrifying moment of truth that his opponents experience. All of his motions are simple and serene; he's barely moving and doing nothing with fists that can fire off like automatic weapons.

He says, "Cut your opponent off in the ring once you understand his habitual path." I was now getting the lesson in making the ring smaller and cutting off my opponent's escape paths. My next goal is to own the ring. Sena taught me that it's like a game of chess.

If you control the center, you control the game. He then broke down how to exploit an opponent's mistakes and ways to evaluate his slight inefficiencies: whether he feels more comfortable going to the right or left. Like a dance, I shuffle forward and back, thinking *my survival is at stake*. It's about my footwork, moving sideways across the ring, locking in by pivoting right before I get to each corner of the ring, reducing the space the opponent can maneuver in, anticipating movements and predicting actions before they happen. *Just calm, confident clear logic*, I tell myself. He'd move to the left, I would then step forward with my left foot and slide with my right foot. It would be the same process again on the right side. I work hard to keep my base strong and my feet grounded with each move.

He's not tired and always one step ahead. Becoming fatigued, I pant hard and lose control of my breath. I now understand how the body starts talking to the mind and the logical concept of mastering my emotions is long forgotten. My intent to stay calm turns to agitation, confidence is replaced with self-doubt—and then, all at once, there's a rush of panic. Keeping him at a distance is a priority. The ring starts to seem very small.

He rushes forward. I'm now facing my biggest fear: the inability to stay calm, trapped in a place where I am physically prevented from leaving. Looking back, the lesson of this morning would be a dress rehearsal for not being able to escape cancer. Backed into a corner, it's easy to lose my senses. I can't think straight. All I need is to remember what Sena told me: "Imagine you have a tool belt strapped around your waist. We are stocking it with tools you can count on using. You will have more options. If it is empty, there is nothing to reach for." Calling on his tools—physical and mental techniques—is everything to Sena.

I get a late life lesson on how situations vary, practicing good timing, and knowing when and how to use the tools of his trade—the fundamental skills of attack and defense that are a prerequisite for life. It's an investment in the proficiency to take care of things yourself, to have the exact tool and to remember to pick it up.

For stocking my tools, I practice the same things over and over again until they become natural: "Don't dwell on your mistakes and keep moving;" "When you are timid—there is a little doubt that creeps in;" "Having confidence is paramount to everything you do;" and "A lot of people will ignore your talent because it makes them feel inferior. They ignore it to make you feel irrelevant."

The physical tools include:
- Keep your chin tucked.
- Elbows in tight.
- Hands up and always bring them back to your chin when you punch.
- When you throw a hook, make sure to shoot the elbow up.
- Parry and counter when your opponent is jabbing and moving to the right; when going to the left, execute a catch and return.
- A way to obstruct your opponent's line of vision is throwing a jab and then dropping down into the pit of the stomach with a punch, coming back with elbows locked.

- The importance of knowing there is a straight line between the chin and target.
- Being defensively responsible after throwing punches, by either moving my head or my entire body to get away from the punches, hinging at the hips, and being explosive.
- Elbows stay tucked when in a boxing stance, to protect the rib cage from incoming blows.

In using tools, accuracy is Sena's preference—being slow and practicing perfect form, as opposed to speed and punching hard but compromising good form. He would repeatedly say to me in his formal, polite style and matter-of-fact tone: "Even when you're tired, don't compromise your form," or "Bring your hand back to your chin every time."

When I was not executing properly, Sena would halt our training to carefully narrate how he used different tools, timing, the proper technique or form by playing a video of his "night before sparring matches." For me, this was like watching the movie *Groundhog Day*. We stood together in the center of the ring, equally fascinated by what we were about to watch. He dissected what had transpired, playing the video in slow motion. We'd see Sena carefully pawing at his sparring partners, allowing his opponent to get overconfident in the ring, just baiting his opponent to throw a punch. Once a punch was thrown, it would never hit Sena. His opponent would then realize he'd been tricked. Sena would then follow with a series of punishing blows. Match after match, it was his way of delivering a crippling message that shattered his opponent's confidence psychologically and physically.

Each sparring match ended the same, with his partner damaged, either on his knees or dazed.

Falling into the corner, the tools were staying calm, switching up the rhythm, moving laterally, or being explosive while rolling and slipping and stepping out. I tried not to let my situation take me off my game plan, but it did. I would experience this exact trapped feeling of reaching into an empty toolbelt with disbelieving eyes when I got the bad news of my cancer diagnosis, medical tests, hospitals, surgeries and found myself in a big-box cancer enterprise while resting in a recliner getting chemo, with a mist clouding my brain. My anxiety spiked and panic set in.

Now things got a little complicated. The corner spot signals a loss of all control for me. I felt the worst possible helplessness, ready to throw in the towel. With my elbows locked, I thought that any place in the ring would be better than where I now stood, like a trapped animal in despair: hopeless. Good fighters understand how to use the corner to their advantage, how to power out of the space to move back to the center, maneuvering the corner and the ropes to tire out their opponent, simply leveraging the space to conserve their energy and then bursting out with an explosive combination.

There's a subtle suffocation that comes with being overwhelmed. The first thought is a desperate call for divine intervention. I reflected back on the exact words that I blurted out the first time I was "placed" in the corner of a boxing ring: "I'm terrified." I covered my eyes as if I could hide myself or become invisible.

Sena showed me an escape blueprint: jab, cross, tuck, jab and then with a slide, step out. I learned that I'm an eternal being and can escape life.

The ceremonial bell rings. There's a one-minute rest.

Round Four

BOXING GLOVES

It was here on Merry Street one January morning that I received a rare gift that I would use as a conduit for strength. More importantly, the gift told me I showed signs of promise. I'd stop dabbling in this boxing hobby as a pure cardio activity and begin an intense investment. From now on, I would no longer be ordinary.

Sena presented me with his own professional lace-up boxing gloves gently worn in a fight by his alter ego, the African Assassin. His perfectly constructed, hand-stitched gloves were of the finest soft cowhide leather with extra-long wrist cuffs for better protection and what felt like a custom fit. If Prada made boxing gloves, these would be the ones in its gallery. Sena acknowledged that it was hard for him to see me training in a franchise gym's cheap steel-gray Velcro boxing gloves meant for a man with large hands. Although they were sold to me as if they were the best gloves on the market, they were oversized and heavy, never properly fit my hands, and gave little wrist support. I had easily settled for them, like other things in my life.

Now I'd move away from the sound of Velcro ripping to the tight, circular double wrapping of the black laces around my wrists, Sena tying a bow and then tap, tap, tapping to indicate I was ready to go. Lace-up gloves have a single lace, criss-crossing the eyelets of each glove to be pulled tight, and then tied in a bow around each wrist. Everything felt less bulky. My training had a new element with these gloves, as they required the help of another person for tying the laces. I knew Velcro gloves were for beginners and these new gloves represented a designation that I might be getting better.

The maker of the gloves, Ramon Arellano, understood that to make something valuable, you have to put your name or face in front of it. Arellano was the owner of a Mexican restaurant equipped with a boxing ring in the center of his establishment, located just behind Hooter's in a neighborhood on the outskirts of Nashville where drug deals take place openly in parking lots. It's an area known for prostitution, tucked behind two shady adult motels, not designed for travelers but for hourly stays; one even advertises the best value rooms in America. My delicately worded questions to trainers about Arellano caused a sense of hesitation, a looking away, as if anything said could be used against them.

The design of the Arellano logo was about elegance over excess, simplicity over complexity. All the elements were at play here: perfect colors, typography, and placement. You'd see the logo and think flawless design: *Boxing Eqmt. Arellano Since '81* on the outside of the wrist and directly above on the knuckles. Four ordinary colors, when placed next to one another, look remarkable. The white leather is a contrast to a rectangle of a vintage, tanned brown leather on the wrist. This was the brown leather of the earliest boxing gloves. A shiny cobalt blue perfectly lines the palm, with black on the exterior of the glove. On the palm, the black strings are threaded through black leather eyelets, and the string then doubles around the wrist with a tie.

My hands were now comfortable, snug in a perfect fit. Not only would the gloves be functional, they'd make a statement. Functionally, these were gloves worn by serious fighters. I ended up leveraging my new gloves in weird ways. Placing them on my table before a virtual client presentation, they'd be a visual reminder that *I had this*. I'd metaphorically climb into the ring for the first official bout of my life against the cancer enemy, feeling as if I was wearing these gloves. They gave me powerful confidence, a belief in myself, a feeling of calm and comfort, got me ready for fight night, and became a sacred symbol to keep my hands up for strength during 11 rounds of chemo and many surgeries. I actually trained with them on my hands during it all.

A catcher's mitt comes to mind when first seeing boxing mitts. They are the first line of defense from wild pitches and hard punches. Both are used to protect the most vulnerable part of the hand, allowing athletes to stay in close touch with the action. There's a beautiful BAM sound that goes with hitting a boxing mitt, similar to hearing a gunshot pitch of 100 mph into the catcher's mitt.

Hitting the mitts while wearing these gloves was one of the big reasons why I came to Merry Street. This was the part I adored most. Sena's bare hands slid firmly into his own black, fingerless gloves attached to the back of thick, durable leather pads that he'd hold for my straight shots and combinations. The prominently placed *African Assassin* name on the wrist of his black mitts was a constant reminder to me of the opponent I was sharing the ring with. This was about precision and measured timing. He set up the flow and rhythm with footwork and smooth combinations, as if arranging seamless musical statements. Watching his arms with the mitts, he could be mistaken for an accomplished percussionist with every beat timed perfectly. His facial expressions and arm movements were at times like a conductor's, suggesting how things should be played and providing feedback. Humming out the rhythm for a few seconds, he determined the tempo, feel, and direction of the beat or punch. He clapped his mitts—BAM-BAM-BAM—to teach me the rhythm.

An hour earlier, with my eyes shut, I had been sitting in my parked car, marking the combo into sections, transitioning with pivots, swivel angles and visualizing myself moving through the space. I had even marked the arm movements while walking around my house the previous day.

Of everything I wanted to do today, this one thing is now most important. He sets up his phone in the corner to capture a video I'd replay later in the day, either to escape a possible mundane reality or to show me how miraculous life had just become. Being capable of absorbing all these combined movements never seemed plausible. It is as odd as abruptly finding myself in a circus tent performing an acrobatic stunt, maybe vaulting onto a horse as part of an equestrian act.

Gesturing me to move forward with his glove, he tells me precisely, "Get into your boxing stance." With my chin tucked, I bend my knees and sink my feet firmly into the canvas, with a balanced fighter's pose. Placing my left foot in front of my right, with my hands to my chin, my focus is on how punching power will be generated from my feet or whipping my hip. My gaze is directly ahead. Like I've learned an ancient art or skill of centuries past transmitted by a master to an apprentice, I had been told I was the only person executing this synchronized routine with elaborate moves in Nashville. It originated in Las Vegas with Sena's Mayweather trainer Rafael Ramos from Puerto Rico, and now it had been passed down to me.

He keeps the mitts close to his body. As a warmup, he calls out the beginning movements of a 40-something punch combination that would one day grow to 82. I feel nostalgic. This could be the last time. The gym would be demolished for a mixed-use office development the next month.

Similar to a dance, the complex combination has codified movements with certain names and expectations associated with each one, such as jab, cross, hook, slip, double roll, trigger, uppercut to the body, pivot, swivel angle, and rock back. Designed for building explosiveness and stamina, each fluid motion is integrated with the next, setting up offensive and defensive maneuvers. There is a logical sequence as each punch is designed to set up the next punch or movement. I held my head high and hung onto each word the day Sena told me that the swivel angles and pivots I had down were advanced movements in boxing.

The exhilaration I'm about to experience is like being in a speeding car on a hilly backroad with my head out the window. The next 34 seconds is the combo, bounded by double lead jabs then in the middle with slips, crosses, uppercuts, hooks, triggers, body shots, swivel angles, pivots and rock backs.

There's a quick 10-second refresh. Like starting a new chapter, he extends his right arm with a bent elbow, guiding me to turn around to a new place in the ring. His facial expressions, eye contact and the way he moves his gloves make it feel like I'm in a real fight with him. I play along and we are right back to the same combination, still focused on technique. We are working on building up speed while keeping accuracy. He tells me to stop drifting to the left and points out my right foot dragging behind my front left foot. I try to keep a relaxed face and relaxed breathing. It's really challenging to do both while I execute movements.

On my hooks, he says, "Elbows in" and then stops to explain. "Your elbows flare out a bit as you throw the punches. Also, they go past that midline between the front and back part of your body. What you want to do is limit the elbow movement to just in front of the rib cage. It means keeping it tight while using your rotational strength in your torso to drive the punches." He no longer gives me the verbal *roll, roll* cue when it's time for a double roll and his arm swings out twice. It's here that I need to go into a deeper squat and lower my body. I've done something to make Sena laugh. On the left and right uppercuts to the body, I'm driving low to the ground.

The double jab at the end of the combination is like the period on the end of a sentence. Sena smiles wide, holds up his mitt for a fist bump and says, "Good work."

I smile, look down, and catch my breath. I have 30 seconds until we start the combination again.

Round Five

DIAGNOSIS

In late Spring of 2018, I had been scheduled for a mammogram. I was reluctant to go. I had disregarded the boob-flattening screening procedure as unnecessary and ridiculous, especially considering how healthy I was from training, Jeet-Kune-Do and boxing.

I also had insider's information into the popular commercial pink ribbon campaign because of my access to a breast cancer scientist who ran her own laboratory with mice at one of the largest academic medical centers. Years ago, while sitting with her at my older son Will's baseball game, I admitted I was at fault and had not had a mammogram. She gazed at me, tilting her head, as if I was gullible and subject to one of the greatest deceptions perpetrated on women of the western world. Her response was to not ever bother getting a mammogram. She shared that the detection of cancer through early screenings was dubious and it put a lot of women through needless stress, and that most biopsies turned out negative, pointing out the potential danger of a needle biopsy causing tumor cell migration—allowing the cancer to spread within the body.

Doing nothing *was* the best plan of action, validated by a scientist with data. I was now smarter than anyone else.

Healthcare is a risky business, with the patient safety problem an open secret among professionals in the industry. Errors are swept under the rug. My daily PR work could have been called "daily secrets the healthcare industry won't tell you—the threat is real." Clients shared emerging hospital threats and errors with me. I lined up media interviews around the what-if scenarios that sometimes became reality. These people were unrestrained about sharing secret details of patient harm and were reliable narrators about deaths due to sloppy errors, accidents, injuries, and infections.

The most common, unequivocal message in working with my clients had been: *A hospital is the most dangerous place in America.* I heard it from nurses, hospital performance watchdog leaders, electronic medical records consultants, cybersecurity experts, and even sitting across a table from the former CEO of one of the largest hospital chains in the country. I knew stunning numbers that showed 200,000 to 700,000 patients die each year as a result of human error.

That I would never be a hospital patient was one of my many framed smug oaths and absolutes in the world. I wanted to stay far apart from a mammogram, not out of anxiety of the unknown or because something would be seriously wrong, but out of complete distrust and fear of the big business of the healthcare enterprise. I feared that I'd be a victim of sloppiness.

The only reason I needed a mammogram now was because of the cosmetic surgery requirement for breast implants. Studying all the elderly gray-haired women sitting around me in a private waiting room, all of us with our legs crossed and wearing pink robes, I noticed their sweet compliance around a harmless procedure that I found painful and made me feel violated. I had scripted the next steps after the mammogram: a retreat to the door, a three-minute drive home from the hospital's breast center, and I'd be back to my PR work in no time. The next day, I'd get a peachy follow-up report and this all would recede and dim in memory.

I received a come-back-in phone call for more images but dismissed the follow-up as just part of healthcare as a business and the need to finance new equipment. Frustrated by the inconvenient disruption, I became even more confident that this was all a big misunderstanding, as if I had walked into the wrong party or had been placed in a high-level math class. Someone, somewhere in the healthcare ecosystem had made a big mistake. It felt as though I was falsely accused. Perhaps it was in the testing process. Or maybe someone was overreacting. Skeptical of the healthcare industry, I thought I had been randomly singled out, with a business objective at play, a cancer quota as part of the healthcare business enterprise strategy.

Motionless and sitting knee-to-knee with a radiologist afterwards, I thought her to be overly dramatic and nervous. I calmly absorbed the strange words about finding tiny deposits of calcium that sometimes indicate the presence of breast cancer. She referred to them as microcalcifications. As I watched her anxiety-ridden face, it felt like the more she talked, the more she just *wanted* to see me cry and feel vulnerable. I didn't panic or experience a loss of control. I wasn't even confused by new medical terms—because I was in complete disbelief.

Of course, I had a clear, concise description of my situation: errors in radiology are unfortunately common. Good doctors are humans and make mistakes. Whether it was human or system-related error, I was pretty confident that negligence was in play as I skeptically scanned the framed medical diploma on the wall. As she talked, I questioned her skills and knowledge. I imagined the bad morning that bled into her work, rushing through things. Or perhaps a corporate bonus was the incentive. Unlike a disadvantaged consumer being lured into a payday loan store, I knew the model of the healthcare industry. I would not be exploited or trapped. I'd be the defector, with others stepping in to take my place. Sitting with her, I felt inconvenienced and quietly angry. The time taken away from my business and workouts weighed on me. I kept my frustration in check. In my universe, things like this didn't happen to me. The radiologist was like an actor with bad form, not following my script.

I thought to myself, *surely if this technology had been around when my maternal great-grandmother was my age, a doctor would have found these so-called calcium deposits in her breasts as well.* She smoked and drank bourbon every day and lived to be 104, and all the other elderly women in my life lived to be 100 or so.

I knew that everything about my health was great. I had made the mistake of stepping into a flawed environment—healthcare. While dismissing her report, I complied with the additional testing. But I didn't lose sleep over the findings, thinking things would soon be cleared up and I'd get an apologetic call any day now, communicating that this was all a big misunderstanding.

All the quantitative data supported that I had an over-abundance of good physical health. My husband's company required an annual biometric screening, conducting laboratory tests that resulted in your personal health assessment profile. If my annual health assessment scores were an IQ test, I would fall into the measurable genius category. I quietly relished nurses' confused expressions at annual checkups. Every year it felt like I was pulling the same harmless, devious prank on a victim. If John accompanied me to an appointment, he seemed to enjoy sitting back and appreciating this game. The nurse would check my resting heart rate, look down to see that the equipment was working correctly, then turn to me, puzzled, questioning that my resting heart rate could really be at 40 or so beats per minute. I would surpass the ideal rate again, placing in the elite health category. I had real-world data to back me up on my premise that my health was something I'd never have to worry about. All I had to do was look around the willful elderly faces at a holiday dinner table to understand that this would one day be me, too.

A month later, I ended up getting the recommended breast biopsy. I was given instructions: *under no circumstances was I to move, not even for a millisecond.* In a prolonged position, where my neck would be twisted by a nurse to the side at a 90-degree angle, I'd be lying on a special table on my stomach with my right breast projecting through an opening in the table; a compression paddle would be used to hold my breast firmly in place, squished. With spasms in my neck and unable to move, it was hard not to think about guillotine executions. I was at the mercy of two indifferent technicians who didn't click, and both were enamored with their cell phones. I practiced my breathing exercises, looked at my lone boob in the X-ray machine and praised it for how well it had served me for feeding my two healthy baby boys. I told myself *you've got this* and wondered out loud what could be taking the doctor so damn long. I asked every 10 minutes if the doctor would be coming soon and communicated how excruciating it was to stay in this position. They insisted they had *just* called the doctor, who was simply upstairs. This happened over and over. Finally, after what seemed like hours, I asked for the phone so that *I myself* could call the doctor. At that point, the two techs shared that they had been dialing the same wrong number this entire time. There were apologies from the doctor when she walked through the door. She then directed a thin needle into my breast to collect a tissue sample.

After the breast biopsy, I couldn't stop the unwanted calls from my doctor saying, "We need to talk..." that went to voicemail. I was annoyed by her insistent urgency. I rationalized that if I didn't call her back, she'd pursue another patient and this just all would go away. Surely, she could see the timing for this wasn't going to work for me. I had just landed a major deal where the new client was waffling between hiring me or a major PR agency. I had a busy schedule of building brands, growing my business and getting my workouts in.

Eventually, I found myself on the phone, faced with what felt like the worst chaos imaginable. I was sweating because of the fast-talking doctor's stream of foreign medical terms: "Biopsy path report: An early stage breast cancer that is triple positive. Breast cancer coming from the ducts of the breast, 1.4 cm, HER2neu positive. To treat cancer—surgery, chemo, plus or minus radiation; hormone blocking pills for the next five years. Surgery comes first. Lumpectomy removes that area. Spend the night in hospital and then remove cancer. Tissue expanders. Lymphoid testing during the surgery. Chemo—a lighter version with hair loss."

My response was: "Good news. It's 1.4 cm and Stage One. That seems tiny and could be cut out. Could we put this off for another six months? I've got so much going on right now." The frustrated doctor said no, that she needed to see me in her office right away.

I slumped back in my chair at an antique marble table that was made to be used outdoors while cutting and arranging flowers. This was the table where I made business deals, crafted clever media placements for corporate clients, and developed sophisticated plans to make people and companies who were nonentities more famous in their industry. It's where I was a phone call or email away from changing people's careers and how they were perceived, building brands to influence sales, landing major business deals, and placing hundreds of published stories for my clients. This table was a representation that I could do anything, anywhere, for anyone.

My daily work here required little equipment, just my own will and guts. It took knowing how to talk to people and understanding in a few seconds how to influence them. A lot of thought went into persuading the media (people I knew well, kind of knew or didn't know at all) via an email message or a phone call to write and publish a story about someone or something. I was securing national attention for people, helping their companies to reposition brands, or positioning their companies for acquisition or investment.

My fundamental belief at the time was that I myself controlled my universe, that I could seriously *will* things to happen or not happen. I proved this certainty to myself daily while sitting at this table. I secured media stories for clients by having quick, friendly conversations with editors and writers. Professionally, I always told my clients, "Hey, it's not if, but when." I was pretty accurate in most cases. The best and closest parking spaces were always empty and waiting for me. I rarely drove the speed limit and sometimes didn't see the rules as applying to me. And I believed that a lot of things that affect most people were not relevant to me or would never occur in my life.

Sitting at my table, I studied the terrifying words on my computer screen and couldn't realize my own story presented there. None of this was plausible. I had been riding the crest of growing my business, and physically I was the strongest I had been in my life, feeling my personal power in a new way. I had started to implement and understand a boxing concept: *If I could access a flow state in the rest of my life, similar to boxing, and be this present in my work, at home, and hanging out with my kids—everything would start to feel more effortless.*

No, this new situation wasn't going to be a good fit for me, not now, not ever. I almost wanted to laugh. I was pursuing something I felt I had deserved—this cosmetic surgery. Now the universe was saying, *I'm sorry, you don't deserve this, but I will give you all of this horrendous stuff instead*—stuff that would take away my health, my mental faculties, my work and the valuable life I was living. This was making me feel vulnerable, having to submit to the healthcare industry.

I was scared, but in a state of hopefulness that I'd iron all this out with the doctor in person.

John picked me up in downtown Nashville from a national Modern Healthcare's *Women in Healthcare* conference for the noon appointment. We looked like any happy couple just out driving in our convertible that summer day. The night before, I was posing for a photo with the CEO of one of the largest health-care systems in the country and pretending life was pretty damn normal and good.

Walking into the cancer surgeon's waiting room, I awkwardly and passively averted eye contact with bald women brushing past me, as if by looking into their eyes I'd be desperately locked together with them. Just like ducking my head while viewing a scary movie scene, this was how I would control my emotions. Making eye contact is about making a connection. One bald woman walking out of the office smiled and seemed to be enjoying her baldness in an exciting way. When I saw her head, my internal conversation firmly said, *"That's not going to be me and I'm not embracing that."*

I approached the receptionist and asked if the doctor was running on time, telling her I needed to go back to an event.

We were led into an awkward, jam-packed room with an examination table and only two chairs. I studied a bulletin board with the doctor's family photos, one from a ski vacation, to better understand how to build my case. I was confident that once the doctor spent time with me, I'd have this situation cleared up and be back to my conference in no time. There was nothing fresh about the room's air. The longer we waited for the doctor, the more I squirmed in my seat, with the room feeling like I was in the rear seat of a minivan packed with clutter, no air conditioning and I was unable to get out. I became dry-mouthed and anxious.

By the time the doctor opened the door, I had forgotten all I was trained to do, all of my breathing techniques and my coaches' advice that your breath *is the number one thing you pull out of your toolbelt in a hostile or uncomfortable situation.* My brain seemed starved from blood flow and oxygen. I expected that the first word out of her mouth would be an apology. Instead, I received what felt like a mechanical recitation from her: the delivery of bad news, straightforward with the word "cancer"; then some foreign medical terms, the need for surgeries, a port and 12 chemo treatments. All of this seemed so casual and accidental. She seemed to be a pro at giving bad news to a patient she had just met, with a career built on women's pain and what felt like a savage ceremony.

Nothing about this situation was evenly matched. Even with her preemptive phone call, I didn't see this blow coming. There would be something obscene, cruel about getting hit this hard. Even with my strong will, sane approach, self-determination, insider's information and good instinct, I realized I wouldn't be able to manipulate this pain, humiliation, loss and chaos. It was unimaginable to me how this doctor, in this strange cramped space, would be dictating my present and future in front of my husband just a few feet away.

I was learning a profound, devastating revelation about my life: I had been well-meaning and deliberate in how I lived my life, trying seriously to be my best self, honoring my family's deeper belief that there was nothing respectable about living with a whiff of fear. Now there was only disillusionment—this was not the destiny I'd hoped for.

While half-listening, I tried to find something that would reveal more about her; I did a head-to-toe assessment. I saw the doctor as an adversary whose sole purpose was to mess up my life. Her precise words around the effects of chemo sounded strangely like she was singing a lyrical song, my own private version, similar to Johnny Cash's rendition of *I've Been Everywhere*. "Persistent symptoms or treatment effects of chemo include the following: hot flashes, muscle aches, blood clots, uterine cancer, cataracts, hair loss, weight gain, nerve pain, scar tissue, decreased shoulder range of motion, chronic pain, lymphedema, neuropathy, low blood counts, decreased heart function, high cholesterol, high blood pressure, secondary malignancy, premature menopause and infertility. Chemo would damage healthy cells, causing loss of memory and cognitive abilities, my hair, eyelashes, and eyebrows. I might expect tooth decay and gum issues, mouth sores, a craving for comfort foods, nausea, constipation, and fatigue most of the time, with potential damage to kidneys, heart, liver, and lungs" …. *and I will have been everywhere, man.*

This was sanity turned inside out. My progress in life was now reduced to the rhythm this doctor had just sung to us like an overused tune. Each word around *chemo's effects* tested the parameters of my entire being. An image of my life and everything I thought I knew about my life snapped: the vulnerability was all playing out. The disintegration of my business, my intellect and good physical health—everything I had worked hard for, accomplishments earned and important to my self-identity— would swiftly go away.

My mind took an abrupt fall into an abyss. My career would have a forgone conclusion: *I have none. Everything ends, so this is how my story ends.* It felt like I crashed to the ground. I experienced a curious sense of time running out, slowing down, multi-dimensional or distorted. Any new joy or hope was now swept away. The jarring suddenness of my life and how "The Lord giveth and the Lord taketh away." How life can go to hell for no apparent reason.

My brain just went offline. My mental self would leave my body. The only dialogue from here out was between John and the doctor. I went from keeping my emotions in check to a devastating psychological paralysis. As if I spoke a primitive language, I could no longer form my words for sentences or questions. I was grateful to John and thought: *This is why you bring someone smart with you to these appointments.* My mind then shifted to going on the run and fleeing to Beirut, where I had been planning a fantasy trip.

I woke up to the doctor's question around my preference of having a double mastectomy or possibly having just the right breast removed. She then tossed around the metaphor of how some women feel wearing mismatched shoes. I opted for the double mastectomy with what little cohesive thought I could muster.

Choking back tears, I started to see an even more terrifying new world: wondering how my husband John would still love me, looking like a corpse with cognitive impairment. And how would I keep my business going and help provide for my family?

The cramped room suddenly shrank even more. My knees didn't buckle, but only because I wasn't standing. In front of the doctor, I had a sudden charley horse, a muscle cramp contraction that locked up, in my left hamstring. It was the hamstring with trauma from when I was 13 years old. Abruptly, I kicked off my beige patent leather Jimmy Choo high heel and stood up on one leg, limping in the confined space, trying not to fall on the doctor, saying "oh, no" and apologizing.

The rest of that day, I hovered in between a place of normalcy and a dense darkness. John dropped me off at my conference, where I sat with women healthcare leaders and listened to what seemed like senseless talks on empowerment. That night, John and I posed for polaroid pictures at a new hotel's penthouse roof-top party as if it were our last night together, me lying across a king-size bed sipping champagne, wearing a cocktail dress and wrapped in a thick robe. No one would have had a clue about what we had just gone through together.

Round Six

"IT'S ALL GOOD"

1977 Nobel Prize winner Ilya Romanovich Prigogine said, "We grow in direct proportion to the amount of chaos we can sustain and dissipate." Prigogine proved that internal self-reorganization can occur after physical and chemical systems are far from the equilibrium. There are messy moments in life that can lead to greater progress. Through navigating something horrendous, you start to see more clearly what has been in front of you all along—what the world is built on—the good and the bad—and that "It's all good," as Royce Fentress likes to say.

As I'd get deeper into trying to master my Jeet Kune Do through boxing, I realized I needed to augment them with something more. I really loved getting better and better by practicing these two things, getting physically stronger, building my skills and knowledge while moving through my limitations. I saw that one thing on my iPhone might help me. For what seemed like a year, I held silent admiration for my lawyer-minister friend Robin's videos of her strength training with a man she called Royce. I asked her to make an introduction. I too wanted this experience that would make me feel deeply uncomfortable, require an intense level of focus and test assumptions about myself. My strength training with Royce was fated to be a meaningful intervention prior to the diagnosis.

Royce is African-American, has the darkest rich brown skin, like obsidian, and brown eyes with hints of blue and hazel. So broad in the shoulders, Royce stands upright and appears more like a lion dressed as a man with a noble, handsome face. He's armed with nothing but confidence. He learned early that life is basically an inner attitude. Always direct, he looks at you squarely and boldly and speaks what he has to say. He has a polite but potentially fierce demeanor. A soldier of football, he knows no barricades. Despair is the emotion felt for the opposing football players who faced Royce. For him, it is business as usual, smashing through his opponents to get to the ball. His eyes tell you everything, as if he is looking inside your head: whether you are progressing forward, need to make a physical or mental adjustment, or are headed to the guillotine. His gruff response, "Off with your head" and "Off with your head again," is for when you have said the wrong thing not just once, but twice. He has set me straight in a blunt harsh tone, sometimes with a smile, but mostly with a gentle straightforward, "Is there a reason *we* are not …," or "Can *we* not do…". He appears to be in his 40s but is older. He loves and respects people who think differently or might be at odds with his thinking.

I had to audition before Royce would accept me on as his client. My tryout process, or "assessments" as Royce likes to call them, lasted a few extra days. Royce smiled, declaring in an exaggerated way, "Who would have *ever* thought I'd be training Kelly?" as if our encounters during the week were inexplicable. He is a former All-American football player, seeing the world through trusted play calls and ways to move the ball down the field. I have zero interest in football. I didn't fit into his narrow scope of clientele. He is all about nurturing elite young athletes, building their mental and physical toughness for entry into the power-house Division 1 programs of football, baseball, softball, and track. Known for helping athletes build a *real* physical advantage, Royce helps them to outthink others on the field, in the moment, and under pressure.

Empowering me physically, he would teach principles that helped me evolve as a person: *you don't want to be brought down by an unexpected tackle; be grateful for the good and the bad; listen to what people don't say; and find a way to eat the elephant*—all while giving me instructions on properly doing pushups, telling me to engage and "screw your hands into the ground." He said that I had "bad energy" when I first met him. He found my words, such as "I can't do that," to be highly offensive.

Simple trivial acts can show we are out of balance in our lives, that we lack simple kindness or basic discipline. Small, everyday actions can tell you everything about how people manage or don't manage their lives, their character, or where they have become sloppy. I learned in my first training audition with Royce—actu-ally, in the first few minutes—that Kelly's approach was broken and would need fixing, and that wasn't easy to hear. All I did, naturally for me, was to kick off my shoes without untying the laces—my routine before stretching and then working out. My untied laces said it all. Royce, with carefully chosen words and a balanced tone, shared that it had been his experience that uni-versity coaches sometimes walk away from considering student athletes when they see them take their shoes off as I had. In one fell swoop, he said I was sloppy or lazy. And it didn't stop there. He pointed out what I thought were inconsequential details and trivialities that said a lot about who I was, like my inability to look at myself in the mirror. He'd position me once a week in front of the mirror and say, "Fall in love with yourself."

He taught me practical ways to stay calm in an uncomfortable social situation, saying, "When you are feeling tearful or vulnerable in a group of people, just hit the reset button and go to the bathroom and regroup." He said things like, "Calm the chatter, do self-talk and self-encouragement and take it in a direction that it needs to go. Do not worry about the guy in front of you."

If I ever faced a hostile situation with someone's arms tightly around me and it felt like there was no way out, what should I do? Royce's demonstration was to show me how remarkably simple some things in life actually are: *all you need to do is completely relax your body, "go noodle" and drop down to the floor to get out of it.*

To help me recalibrate with my challenging client, Royce said: "If these guys are saying negative things, look at Kelly first, then rectify their concerns. Running from it is not the answer. If we can fix Kelly, we can fix situations with your clients. When you are dealing with multiple leaders in one company, make sure you pave the road so you are the lighthouse." In response, I would look deeply at my business—my guidelines, standards, check points and protocols. In managing criticism, Royce would teach me the power of listening. "Listen and be cool. Tell yourself: I am here to help solve problems, I will listen and respond and put together a solution. Don't let this one client play inside your head. Discipline your emotions. You are giving this guy energy and making him bigger than he is … it will take you on a roller coaster ride." And he'd say, "You got the juice. He's got the title. You are not going to keep throwing crap at me—I'm throwing it back. You don't need to be bitchy, but you don't need to bite your tongue either."

As a result of training with Royce, I began to coach myself every day around my difficult client. I would follow a step-by-step process so my client meetings would go smoothly. It started with me slowing down my speech, saying things to show respect and knowing I am in control. Then there'd be a demonstration of empathy, not interjecting and listening carefully. Next, I'd identify the problem, avoid blame and resolve the problem by talking about processes and best practices to see how to get the best outcomes and identify where there were disconnects.

What I started learning physically in working with Royce was the relationship between body and mind, the power of breath, and how to engage muscles and connect with the earth. And most importantly, that our beliefs have a lot of power; they tell us what to trust.

Royce would say, "We take our breathing for granted. If I held you underwater, you'd appreciate your breathing." "Really exaggerate your breathing," Royce would tell me as I descended into a Cossack squat while holding weights. Learning a movement to help build range of motion, I'd descend with the majority of my weight on one leg and the other leg straight out to the side, heel on the ground with toes pointing up in the air. "The beautiful thing about exercise is, the body tries to control the mind, but you can control the body through the breath."

***

The word cancer had barely been spoken to anyone. I planned to use my strength training with Royce as distance from my diagnosis a month ago, in an effort to snap back to feeling a sense of normal. Yet my mind had been changed. I was walking into a warehouse gym that was equipped like a CrossFit gym—including two squat racks, dumbbells, barbells and cable machines, with an entire wall covered with college flags brought in by clients— but I was collapsing in the opening seconds, sucked under by what felt like permanent defeat, a loss of control, and an inability to maintain my defenses. Everything about this workout for the next hour turned into just keeping my composure. Royce would demonstrate each movement he wanted. I'd work hard to make his vision real. Presenting your best self and making that slight stretch above your skill set is how you naturally want to show up with Royce.

At moments I'd bite my lips, force my eyes shut or touch my eyes to recover from any visible tears as I tried to hinge at the hips, balancing on one leg while holding a heavy dumbbell close to my thigh and connecting my toes to the ground in what is called an RDL. As I was pushing my hips up high and holding for hip thrusts, or getting low and holding my chest up while doing kettlebell squats, or landing jumps onto a plyo box platform, I was trying not to cry.

I felt as if crying in front of Royce was not allowable. This was the man who said that when I find myself in an uncomfortable situation, I could politely leave and go to the bathroom to "fix my face." When I displayed bad energy, he would say to me, "Go inside and fix yourself." Or when I was training and I'd had a bad day, he'd tell me, "Put your feelings in your pockets." If trauma from an old injury caused me to complain about my hamstring locking up, he would say, "You have all your feelings up in your hamstring." I quickly realized it was not my situation, it was just *me* who needed fixing. It's about having the ability to rise above. He had disciplined his mind and emotions to an art and regularly reminded me, "Your head, your mood is your property." And "Don't let anything come into here," as he drew a circle around my face with his index finger.

No one is prepared for the mental strength of Royce. Nothing would ever rattle this man's cage. I knew he was the master at managing emotions just like I understood that I woke up breathing. It's unthinkable that Royce could be erratic or reckless. Watchful of everything, he keeps his inner self untouchable from the everyday, from incidental contaminations that flow around and seem to touch the insides of everyone else. This former football player was known for his mighty fighting capabilities, fighting his own team members his freshman year of college to get out of a humiliating hazing talent show. Lying in bed at night as a child, he grew accustomed to the screams for help of drunken men drowning in a rock quarry behind his house. Now his blind dying father lived with him.

It was never my plan to cry in front of Royce. I had a sense of relief, thinking I had successfully made it through the workout and controlled my emotions. I was sitting upright on the floor with my legs stretched out in a relaxed middle-split position, with my toes to the ceiling, when a peculiar thing happened that caused me to burst out crying. After training, Royce typically walks around the gym putting equipment away while talking to me about something important. But on this day, he sat on the floor and faced me eight feet away and joined me in stretching. In this deserted gym, he mirrored me in the exact same stretch. I paused to take heed of Royce's dancer-like flexibility, turnout and graceful movement, confirming my silent belief: Royce could have been a dancer had he not found football. Not another soul was to be seen and there were no distractions or props.

I felt my chest tighten. On overload, I pictured a devastating loss of all of my progress and saw a new future in which I might be reduced to something I no longer recognized. I had been tripped up by my imaginative powers and denial. The order of my world no longer made sense and I didn't know how to proceed. People die suddenly. I didn't know what to expect any longer.

Feeling hopeless and helpless, I continued to cry while reaching my left arm up and over my head to gaze at the ceiling, then facing my right knee, then placing hands in the center with my face down, easing my chest forward and maintaining a straight spine as I walked my hands out (anything to hide my face). Tears running down my face, all I could think about was how I had slipped down in Royce's estimation. It was one of the most uncomfortable situations. I then became more worried for Royce and his feelings, wondering if he had ever been face-to-face with a crying woman.

I questioned myself: *Did it make sense to tell Royce?* Yes, I decided. He might ask one day why I stopped training or what happened to my hair and body. We were two figures facing each other on the floor with legs stretched out to each side when I told Royce the news about my visits to the doctor and nutritionist.

There was nothing ambiguous or blurred about what took place next in this time and space. It was about my own destiny. I sat there motionless. He began showing me what *not* to do. It started with his physical response that instantaneously pulled me from a sense of loss to *let's get beyond the pain and win this*. I was silent, suspended in a way, with his eyes staring back at me. These eyes weren't stunned or sad. He didn't adjust his position. He looked at me squarely and spoke: "You've known about this and today we are not going to have a pity party." He'd be deliberately calm, with no emotion. Here I received one of my life's biggest gifts: finding a deeper reserve of self from a man who sees the world through winning and a trusted playbook. He shared how pity is a destructive enemy, draining you of mental and physical strength, keeping people stuck in a dark place.

For Royce, the great enemy of winning is pity or worry. He'd tell me, "Worry is the thief of peace and joy." And "The mind is a muscle and you have to be careful of your thoughts." Or "When you are not one hundred percent, someone or something will get the best of you." He wasn't going to comfort me with expressions of sorrow, enabling me to stay stuck. Any form of pity—either through a demonstration of words or feelings—would not improve my situation. He was pragmatic in his approach: it's about facing the truth and not being driven by fear.

The next part followed as if he were saying: *I shall tell you everything you need to know. You will not have to worry about anything.* He'd be sharing "back-pocket information," a phrase he uses with his young athletes to set them apart from others—information not intended for sharing—to help me face what would be the greatest fight of my life. This marked the beginning of my self-organization to navigate a way out of the unpredictable and random chaos of breast cancer. He gave me the gift of telling me about hardship and sharing valuable lessons in how he learned to manage his life.

Amidst my uncertainty, sitting on the floor of this gym, Royce helped me define priorities and start making decisions. I saw my priorities: my marriage, my kids, and my health. Right there, everything became about doing what I wanted to do and what was right for me and my immediate family. My self-preservation kicked in. I knew I wanted to keep my mind and body in fighting shape. With chemo and surgeries approaching, I'd need to focus on my conditioning, become mentally tough, and surround myself with trainers endowed with physical and mental assets beyond those of ordinary men. My strategy was to have the best possible "good endgame," and that meant having non-complicated surgeries with quick recoveries and minimal downtime.

Combined with mastering the mind, I knew that the best-conditioned athlete owns the advantage. In learning about my opponent, I would need to move and dictate the pace of the fight. I would be the underdog. My focus was to minimize my risk with a healthier body through the right nutrition before the surgery, which would lead to a quicker recovery. I would heal myself through eating. I'd need to find ways to give my body energy with a clean diet, creating a strong immune system, exercise and meditation.

To help me transition my thinking around giving up food and drinks I craved, Royce referred to my new way of eating as: "It's a new lifestyle." For stocking up on my energy, emotional reserves and finding new coping mechanisms around self-care, he said, "Fuel your morning with water, gratitude, stretching and meditation." I'd need to become more inwardly-directed and start bringing a more gentle, caring attitude toward myself. I took Royce's vantage point to manage what seemed impossible and undeniable. I used his philosophies and training rituals to get better in my boxing and help overcome my cancer.

What Street Your Parade is On?
I listened to Royce's approach to sharing personal information. He'd say, "I don't tell people the name of the street I hold my

parade on"—which translates to: *When you have something going on, be relentlessly guarded with what you share and with whom.* I could name the people I wanted in my corner, a central command "war room," and trusted advisors to provide collective thinking. This was a foundational philosophy to guide my communications about my breast cancer diagnosis and made me feel that I could manage how people approached me.

The Queen: It's a Hill

I'd bow to the queen, but not to cancer. Royce introduced me to this particular Queen, a hill who "makes you bow," makes you conscious of the ups and downs and your lack of discipline.

Part of my approach for managing breast cancer was to use Royce's back-pocket information on how to run "The Queen," as he calls it. The Queen is a 137-meter-long grassy hill with an alarmingly steep grade in East Nashville's Shelby Park. The experience made me understand: *You don't have to like me, but you will respect me.* The first few steps would teach a straightforward understanding of order and class systems: *I am inferior and she is superior.* It was about honoring and acknowledging her authority, and showing humility when you get to the top. Everything should be deliberate and with the intention of showing special respect. The Queen is about improving your mental and physical power in what could be an overwhelming situation, testing your own fight-or-flight response, and about dealing with one difficulty at a time.

Before charging up the high ground, it is like meeting an actual queen, simultaneously feeling nervous and excited. Royce's first instruction was: no matter what, *never look up at the top of the hill.* He told me I'd regret it. I was to stay focused on my breath and look only at the grass directly in front of my feet. And when I started to struggle, I heard him say, "Listen to the birds or the wind, or in your mind go to that beautiful place you want to go, or get a mental picture of that future person you strive to be."

I started at the bottom with my back to the flat winding road, the Cumberland River and slow barges. The idea is not just to reach the top as quickly as possible, but to appreciate the position and power of the Queen by dropping down and doing push-ups or shadowboxing after climbing a hill that doesn't seem runnable. For the descent, I was told to simply walk down to the bottom. I then returned to the Queen and sprinted back up, reached the top and did push-ups or shadowboxing, walked down—and repeated, over and over again. I started with four or five intervals and then increased to 45 minutes.

Standing at the bottom of the Queen, my intention was to follow his directions literally. The smallest glance up to the crest was overwhelming and made me sway. The easiest part would be starting. My heart raced bounding up the hill, and I'd find my immediate rhythm on the climb and watch the blades of grass, tiny purple flowers and clover pass by directly in front of my toes. In just a few seconds, I gasped for air, my legs were heavy and my rhythm no longer existed. The grade of the hill triggers panic and self-doubt. By the time I could see limestone sticking out of the ground, my inner critic was saying, *there's no way. Or remind me, why are you even doing this?* I turned to focus on my breath. In my head, I could hear Royce's words: "Let the mind override the body." I continued to climb, feeling her wrath as I was only halfway to the top.

The slope got steeper and it felt like I was climbing a vertical wall. I'd lose my momentum and the angle overpowered me. I concentrated on Royce's words, *A strong body was not made in comfort. When it starts to burn, tell yourself you want more.* I'd put one foot in front of the other and follow Royce's precise instructions. I'd make it to the top and feel lucky to shadowbox. My walk down was all about regrouping for the next climb and mind management.

Next time, I'd get myself out of the way, follow Royce's exact approach and attack what was in front of me. I'd plan to take each of my six surgeries, the six different six-week spans of recovery time, the long four weeks of the drains with long tubes inserted into my breast area, the eleven chemo treatments, the weekly blood draws from my port, and all the related side effects just as if I were running the The Queen.

Visualization

Royce encouraged me to set my intention and visualize the outcome: how I wanted to feel and how I wanted to look two years and five years from now. Early in our training, he demonstrated the power of setting expectations and "putting it on your brain thread." I'd stand at a free-throw line with a basketball. Eyes closed, I made effortless baskets after visualizing the ball making it into the net. He showed me the power of *expecting* that I could actually land new and unimaginable business contracts. Months after making a presentation to a prospective client's CEO and leadership team, where I was way too blunt about their company's brand, and not hearing back from them, Royce reminded me to follow up—because, "it was going to happen." And it surprisingly did. He was 100 percent confident that I would arrange a visit with the musical artist Lizzo when she came to Nashville—simply because "I had already put it out there in the universe." Once again, Royce was right.

I was determined to train with Royce as much as possible leading up to my first surgery on September 24. He had a strict "six weeks of no working out after surgery" policy for his clients that I would follow. I decided getting as strong as possible would speed up my recovery.

During our time of intensive training, he shared videotapes of me doing pull ups with a band, Arnolds with hand weights or pulling a heavy sled across the gym. These would be powerful visuals for me to study at the hospital to tell myself to stay strong.

Round Seven

PRE-FIGHT

Investors bought up just about everything in the Merry Street gym's neighborhood. The gym had closed and its boxers had moved on. This was the place where I shared my diagnosis with Sena and Christy. Now, 60 hours before my scheduled surgery, I'd look around at what most people might consider a dreadful, lonely, dirty place—Randall's gym—and experience a serene Zen-like feeling, even as I knew parts of my body would soon be removed.

Randall's newly opened boxing gym, more of a secret gym, had dusty plastic storefront windows covered in thick, black, metal bars. It was at the corner end of a rundown strip mall, surrounded by fast cash storefronts, next to a worn-down Dollar General store and a Rent-a-Center. It was without electricity—no lights, no fans or air conditioning—and at the time, no running water or bathroom. Every heavy bag, piece of equipment, and even the Olympic 16 x 20-foot red, white and blue boxing ring with its perpetual central creak under the padding, was a hand-me-down from the Merry Street gym.

It was here that my soul was in perfect order. As if it was intended and how it should be. In Randall's new gym where it didn't seem possible to breathe. Where some of the time, I'd walk into darkness. Where not a soul was to be seen around this gym's deserted shopping center. My thoughts were not scattered, and I was not startled by what I was getting ready to go through.

On this night, anchored by my pre-fight strategy, I started seeing myself in a state of progress rather than as a mess. It felt as if I'd done something miraculous. I was no longer crawling, operating from a place of fear and allowing it to direct my decisions. While studying my form in the mirror and jumping rope, I realized my training had toughened me up, my body was stronger than ever, I had conquered my flaws, and mentally, I had my approach in place. My training taught me how to stay calm and controlled and not use any energy that is not necessary.

After jumping rope for 10 minutes straight without tripping once, the reality set in—I'd come a long way. I was pleasantly surprised that all the good stuff I had been doing for myself to get through the anguish of the past two months had paid off.

Exactly two months since my surgeries had been scheduled, I was in a boxer's meditative training state as it related to my work-out and the trauma my body was about to endure. Frozen in this moment, the pieces of the jigsaw puzzle found their correct positions. I had found peace and contentment. I knew I was ready to be in the ring. My eyes and body adjusted to something better. My body showed that it would not betray me. I had abandoned my established ways of being. Getting my body clean would be perfectly timed with surgery and chemo.

After winding up my rope and putting it in my bag, I shared a key fact with Sena: On Monday morning, I'd be getting my boobs cut off. This would be our last workout for six weeks.

Dust was suspended in the air so thick that it was tough to breathe with my heart rate up. Standing in the middle of the ring during a mitt combination, I stopped to ask Sena if this place was comparable to the Bukom gym where he trained as a college student after a 45-minute bus ride at 3 a.m. from Accra. Sena told me no, that was not the case. "The ocean is right there," he said, pointing to an empty parking lot. Right outside, goats were piled up and their hides were burned in open fires. "So many goats' hides each day," Sena reflected and said with a smile, "I wondered if there were any goats left in Ghana."

From the beginning, things Sena did at Randall's gym told me it might not be safe. He greeted me in the parking lot, locked the gym door behind us and, in the ring, while managing combinations and holding both the mitts and a steady-eyed gaze at me, he scanned the parking lot past my head as if a predator was on its way, seeing and sensing movement outside his direct line of sight.

Before the sun came up or in the evening, the only light was from Sena's flashlight. He met me in the parking lot and then stood at the front door. "Give it some time, your eyes will adjust to the darkness and you'll start to see your surroundings," he quietly said. In the early mornings, like a statement of law, Sena would say, "Start jumping rope. When you are finished, the sun will come up." He started his stopwatch while saying, "ten minutes." This was how we started every training session—by jumping rope for seven, eight, or ten minutes. When he precisely emphasized "Time!"—the morning sunbeams poured through the window. Like an apparition or a demonstration of God's will, he stood in front of the window, a silhouette outlined in a luminous, opaque haze.

After receiving the cancer diagnosis, I was terrified and overwhelmed, as if my breath had been taken away. I shrank into a private misery of doubt, trying so hard to keep my eyes forward, with my face in a boxer's neutral gaze. Meditating about my upcoming plight and counting down the days to facing the knife, I knew that the body parts that defined my femaleness—the ones that emerged way too early, causing uncomfortable attention but later critical to motherhood, equipping me to feed my healthy sons—would be carried away for good. At first, I was flailing wildly with acute determination to get my body ready for the *fight*.

In preparation for the events of the next six months, I'd put myself through the ultimate test of endurance before my fight. I went into extreme preparation to achieve something big that required important work and discipline. I'd be getting into fighting shape—preparing my mind and body for the battle with cancer, just as the boxer prepares for possible cumulative blows, pain and major damage in a full match with twelve rounds. Knowing my opponent's notoriety around the violence of his fights, I didn't want to get brought down by a single blow.

I'd be shaken to my core as I was getting "clean" overnight, learning and practicing a new lifestyle that would be radically different. I felt like I was barely functioning, free-falling, while simultaneously in a state of disorientation. My body and mind were lethargic and I had headaches for the first time while having the worst food cravings of my life. I'd started off in what felt like quicksand, experiencing a crash of body and mind and a real sense of anguish. For more than a month, my mind felt as if it was choking on heavily polluted air. My mental and physical abilities were slowed to a crushing crawl. I was in a thick mental haze, comparable to the worst hangover that could not be shrugged off. The exhilarating, euphoric rush of caffeine, alcohol and sugar was replaced by nothingness.

Physically, I could see change. I lost 10 pounds overnight that I would have guaranteed could never come off my body, no matter how hard I tried. I looked lean and ripped. A few days into my new lifestyle, Sena told me I was a better boxer than previously. Royce communicated immediately how my energy had changed. Courtesy became more relevant in my life. I noticed I was a better PR professional, listening more intently to my clients and securing more publicity for them than ever before. Voices of doubt that I had carried with me like a heavy backpack went away. My critical judgment of myself and others, sometimes harsh, left me. I became a kinder, more engaged wife and mother. I started to see grace all around me as my state of mind changed. I hadn't felt at home in the world, but now I did.

My change in lifestyle took faith and perseverance. I was feeling the natural and beneficial reactions of my body trying to detoxify, heal, and balance itself. I would eventually experience positive, natural discharges of energy that included clearer thinking, more energy, and stamina. By being intentional, I was already changing direction. I was finding self-respect through this intense boxing training and disciplined eating. I started getting in touch with a stronger sense of my self-worth. For the first time, I had a gentle, caring attitude toward myself.

During the two months of preparation, I told myself: *I know you don't want this. I know you don't deserve this. But this is your path. Work with the path, don't fight it. All the fighting will get you stuck.* I'd tell myself to have patience, courage, and a commitment to see myself through the changes. As a result, I started to reconnect again with my own value.

In two ways, my pre-fight plan would not be unlike Rocky Balboa in that tenement flat, waking at 4 a.m., cracking five eggs into a blender and downing a glass of raw egg whites and yolks. Rocky knew he needed protein. I too would eat things that might not be a pretty sight and I'd take on new routines as if my life depended on it. Right away I had to strengthen my immune system, increase iron intake, support my digestion and inflammatory markers with a goal to alkalize my blood, calm my nervous system and increase my Yang energy to balance estrogen and progesterone. Japanese warriors ate umeboshi plums before going into battle. I'd eat them every day, along with a diet of fermented solid bean paste for miso soup, Japanese sea vegetables such as wakami, dulce and arame, lotus and burdock roots, 20-plus vegetables a day, adzuki beans, plant force liquid iron, liquid chlorophyll, aloe vera juice, royal maca with DIM, groats and dandelion, kukicha, mushroom and green teas. My morning breakfast routine involved slicing vegetables for boiling water, creating a miso soup from a paste.

I would find an unconventional way of managing the powerlessness and fear through a diet and lifestyle prescribed by an authority on healing the body through macrobiotic food.

Meat, sugar, poultry, dairy, caffeine, alcohol, eggs, bread, and carbonated beverages would go away. Raw vegetables were forbidden, along with tomatoes, potatoes, eggplant, and peppers. I was to avoid vegetable juices, alcohol, sparkling mineral waters, cold drinks, and sugared or stimulant beverages. I would cook only with gas, use pots and pans of stainless steel, ceramic or cast iron. All my new meals were prepared via boiling, steaming, or sautéeing with oil. I trained myself to learn a new way of slicing, moving away from the old haphazard way of chopping vegetables. I'd need to incorporate new behaviors around chewing my food slowly, telling myself repeatedly *my body is in the healing space*, while thinking about and visualizing how each bite would heal me. I would take so many supplements that I felt like a witch doctor.

***

My pre-fight boxing training plan for cancer had taken a hard blow one early Friday morning in mid-May. After running hill sprints up to the top to reach Sena on Merry Street, in between the rusty RV and medical supply truck, staring down at the long center crack, I was trying with each sprint to improve my earlier time. I stopped at the top when I heard his voice say, "Time!" and we walked down the hill together. Then Sena looked down and, in a soft tone, began to share his news by saying, "So, Kelly." He'd be unexpectedly leaving tomorrow for a month or so of training in Houston to get some distance from an unraveling relationship. It was the fastest and best solution.

Unexpected goodbyes for me are the toughest kind. With my world turned upside down, I had wanted to keep my sense of normal and lean into the enormousness of his profound self-assurance for inspiration, hoping that it might rub off on me during this preparation period. I was certain that I'd never see him again and I thought we were saying a final goodbye. When someone dropped out of my life, I sometimes resorted to blaming myself, thinking I might have done something wrong. I was trying to be pragmatic here. It was evident my training with him had an expiration date. He was a transient force, moving on in pursuit of his pro boxing dreams.

I was happy for Sena, considering that this might be the one thing to propel him to the top of the boxing hierarchy, but I hated abrupt goodbyes like this one. I'd return to my car out of breath and think about how we don't realize when it's the last time for doing something until there are no more times left. The reality was that no other trainer would ever be able to instruct the 40-plus, ever-growing mitt combination with me. And, as I age, I wouldn't be able to do it forever. I'd miss how he greeted me in the mornings: a formal etiquette, broad smile, saying with a nod of the head, "Good morning and welcome," followed by, "Quickly, let's get to work." This unmistakable greeting was coming from the same man who, at the beginning of a boxing match or when sparring, would have a distinctive salutation for his opponents. Just as he would respectfully welcome me, he would look each opponent in the eyes before each match, extend a pleasant smile and kindly say, "There will be blood…and it won't be mine." He was simply sharing the inevitable in a happy way. A larger truth. He knew the effectiveness of communicating a succinct story and how it could have a simple, devastating cause and effect. The simpler the story, the more it would stick.

For the next few weeks, I'd play back how much I had learned from a 26-year-old who had randomly shown up in Nashville. He'd taught me a boxing rule that I'd adopt for my new life in fighting with cancer. *When slipping or rolling to avoid a punch, you have to physically lean forward into your opponent or the threatening situation and not away, making you well-grounded and better positioned to follow up.* Leaning away affects your balance, keeps you in the line of fire and puts you in an even worse situation. I'd learn a trick to obstruct my opponent's line of vision and just drop down into the pit of the stomach with elbows locked. Being defensively responsible would be important for the next few months.

The drills he set up after throwing punches involved either moving my head or my entire body to get away from the punches my opponent would throw back at me. He showed me how to exploit an opponent's mistakes; how to evaluate the slight inefficiencies of an opponent, whether he feels more comfortable going to the right or left; how to parry, a lovely efficient slight swat down of the hand as a defensive move when an opponent throws a jab or cross; and how to parry and counter when an opponent is jabbing and moving to the right; and then, when going left, how to execute a catch and return.

And then my friend and boxing coach left.

Two days before my double mastectomy surgery in September, I had my last boxing training with Sena for two months. Off to Las Vegas, he trained at Floyd Mayweather's gym and returned in late November for his December fight outside of Nashville. While he was away, he sent frequent encouraging notes, saying things like: "I know you'll come back stronger and better!" or "Wishing you the best and sending you lots of positive vibes."

***

The next Monday morning, at the Merry Street gym without Sena, I'd stare down at my four fingers and thumb spread out wide and experience an uncustomary, intricate and elegant form of hand wrapping taught to me by a woman who is arguably one of the most important figures in women's boxing. This would be my tiny, valuable lesson in self-sufficiency—how one can be extraordinary in doing any common practice, like protecting the fighter's hand, a practice that has been around almost as long as the beginning of boxing. She didn't say a word, but it was made clear she wouldn't be wrapping my hands after today. I'd need to pay close attention to her rapidly weaving the wraps back and forth half a dozen times in the air, then placing the giant padding of wraps on my knuckles, with my thumb holding it in place, coming around a few times to cover it, slipping the thumb out, twisting the wraps around the wrists, then weaving around the inside of the fingers. I would try hard to memorize her technique while questioning: *why have I not been wrapping my own hands before?*

I'd spend three days a week for the next two months with Christy Halbert, Ph.D., author of a book that passed down boxing concepts typically reserved for the elite boxing establishment. She had coached the 2012 women's boxing Team USA that won two medals (a gold and a bronze) and gained legitimacy for women in the sport. The night before my first session with her, I'd get her up to speed by sharing recent videos of me hitting the mitts with Sena, offering her immediate clarity of what her time with me would look like. She offered me feedback such as, *good movement forward: pushing off the back foot: extension of the punch is good. However still turning the punch over a little early. :-)*

My training with Christy was about her gathering evidence around the state of my form and logically correcting technical deficiencies, things that Sena had noted, but we hadn't had the chance to work on. She offered a precise, kind ease in her instructions, after making simple analogies and metaphors that would promise fast, positive results. She instructed me to "whip my right hip like Elvis" when throwing a cross; or to "have footwork like a cat's paws grasping" when going up and down in the ring to help me to maintain equal footing distance; and which foot to push off with when moving forward and when moving back. I would know more about keeping my balance as I was moving in the ring.

Standing eight feet away, while I was ready in my boxing stance, she'd throw a basketball at my face to help me with explosivity, arm extension, and the timing of when to turn my wrist. I'd punch it back to her with a jab or a cross. She put a 6-foot pipe on the floor for footwork drills to correct my too-wide boxing stance and to help with my footwork stepping, letting me see that I was incorrectly dragging my back foot when moving forward.

My training with Christy would help me to further develop my pre-fight plan—applying the science and strategic principles behind boxing to have physical strength, endurance, and power. I'd start to choreograph what would be my pre-fight ritual leading up to my surgeries and chemo: things like jumping rope, shadowboxing, and hitting the speedbag.

Jumping Rope

Jumping rope is how I kicked off all my workouts, and it took my endurance and agility to a new level. On the spot, Sena would give me lightning-speed instructions along with a demo, followed by the playback request: "Ok, now let's see it," without giving me a moment's notice to think about it. Though seemingly impossible and laughable at first, I would turn around, surprisingly execute, and be proud of the new trick I had just added to my skipping repertoire.

When I first jumped rope, I felt the most overwhelmed, with fear of falling short, that expectations somewhere weren't being met. I couldn't find my breath, hated the fact my choices were limited to jumping up and down and turning my wrists, and I wanted to flee. My approach was all wrong, as if I was in a battle with the rope. After a minute, two minutes or three minutes, my legs felt heavy. I'd hit a dark uncomfortable place, sucking in air and trying desperately to keep from tripping on the rope. I'd hear my inner critic tell me: *PICK UP YOUR FEET*. I'd wince at the burning sensation if the cable rope ever abruptly smacked my bottom. Each day I held up Sena's personal story against mine. I heard on occasions how he skipped rope for hours with weights on his ankles in a competition with his uncle back in Ghana. I surely could do this for three, seven or ten minutes. He'd closely monitor and be quietly disappointed if I'd accidently trip on the rope after saying "Time!" As I jumped, I stayed focused on not tripping while increasing my time. Because of this, I just kept getting better.

Jumping rope with Sena taught me to hang tight in what felt like a spinning-out-of-control situation with my breathing, the movements of the arms and jumping of the feet. I'd be forced to go inside my head, relax, keep a focused gaze and just be with Kelly. There'd be no room for my inner critic or ego. I'd have the right form so that I didn't trip or exert more energy than necessary. A byproduct would be learning how mental ease was controlled with the coordination of breath.

Taking time to study my form in the mirror, I'd feel gratified by my meditative focus and ability to control my breath and slow it down when the amount of time jumping seemed overwhelming. With improved coordination, I'd take it up a notch to jumping jacks and sideswipe criss-crosses, then to complex jump rope routines with "double-unders." The pinnacle of my jump rope routine would be flipping front to back while continuing to skip rope.

Getting into a rhythmic flow for a straight ten minutes began feeling like the norm. I was focusing on my breath and synchronizing my mind and body to be in the present, on most days without ever tripping over the rope.

I'd learn to masterfully jump rope like a *real* boxer after hearing Christy say, "whip each hip to the corners of the gym." Then she introduced a concept that seemed so wildly strange to me that I declined at first. She asked for me to get into the center of the ring with my rope and jump. Jumping rope in the ring would become my new space for meditation and making contact with my power.

Shadowboxing
Shadowboxing is doing whatever you please, in free form, to demonstrate your power and imagination with zero distractions. It's complex and simple. In a freestyle form, you do whatever you please while physically, it tests your explosiveness, form, speed, footwork, head movement and ability to stay comfortable while moving. It's about staying relaxed while putting together

rhythmic combinations for attack and defense. I'd need to understand spatial awareness and how to evade punches from an imaginary opponent to see myself as a certain fighter.

I'd be told one of boxing's most important principles while shadowboxing in the ring: *Focus on you. You know your power.*

At first, I felt like a painter with a limited imagination in front of a blank canvas. Or as if I had been asked to do a naked improv dance as part of an art project. I was so tight and rigid when asked to shadowbox in an empty ring that I would just freeze. My sense of wonder, curiosity, confidence, and imagination that were my assets as a kid had diminished over time.

Christy would help me to overcome an overwhelmed feeling and find my confidence, my own personal style, flow and power. She would ask me, "What is your signature combination?" to help me take it from intimidation to excitement. She'd talk to me about how vulnerability can be an asset. "Allow yourself to be vulnerable to create openings. You create the openings and opportunities, be willing to throw a punch, be vulnerable, act first—then when you do, effective things happen in the ring, then the opening to the body is available." I'd be told in the ring, "Sometimes a threat is disguised as an opportunity."

Shadowboxing allowed me to step out of my routine of self-judgement and self-editing to think about taking risks, creating what was my own experience. I'd work at different levels to see what emerged from my center. I'd later get into the ring thinking about the structure I was asked to set up, how to focus on being fluid, my direction, slipping, rolling and shifting levels and tempo—all while trying to make each movement unpredictable. Constantly moving my feet laterally, shifting, retreating, taking quick step-offs at a rapid pace while staying mentally focused on an invisible opponent, I'd find shadowboxing to be one of the most grueling workouts physically and mentally.

Speedbag

I had skirted around the speedbag in the corner of the gym, avoiding it like a bully. Visually and audibly, in a clear and precise fashion, with my fists in space, the speedbag told me I wasn't enough. I let this small, leather, air-filled 6 x 8-inch bag anchored to a platform get inside my head.

Irritation is what my face first showed when Sena told me to hit the speedbag, and on most days to keep me comfortable he kept it out of our workout. My first experience left a lasting impression of frustration. I felt physically challenged trying to accurately strike the speedbag, yet I was unable to keep it continuously moving straight. With my hand wraps loosening, finding a rhythm in striking the bag left me feeling stupid, clumsy, and awkward. It was also about me feeling uncomfortable in what I saw as an out-of-control situation. The bag flying around chaotically, not coming back to me, just magnified that safety for me is about having everything under control.

"Make invisible bread plate-size circular motions with your fists, elbows resting on a high countertop while hitting the bag with the meat of your hand," said Christy. Based on her simple instructions, I saw a miracle—becoming proficient on the speedbag my first day of training with her. She'd say, "Make the bag adjust to you." In her short instructions, what I heard was a multitude of things: *when you find yourself in a situation that isn't working for you, make it work, figure it out, look for patterns, make the situation adapt and adjust to you. You can change the situation you are in, change the situation to suit you, you are the ultimate controller, and use your power to move things in any direction you so choose.* Christy would continue by saying, "Sometimes we make adjustments, other times we need to stick to our game plan and allow the process to work. And then other times we force the bag to make the adjustment to us."

I'd start with my breath to gain control of the situation. When hitting the bag for a long time, I'd intensely connect my feet to the ground, with a focus more on my legs, less on my arms, moving in a circular motion.

Later I'd be able to hit the speedbag and see it as my soulmate. It revealed how I had told false narratives about myself, showed me how I felt shame when actually I was doing something fairly well. It showed my strengths: endurance, power and upper body strength. I'd fall in love with the split-second timing of the sound and visual movement of the lightning speed of the bag coming forward and back.

I wanted to be *that* smart fighter—the one who, while training my body, trained my mind. I wanted to be ready for that first punch. My concentration would be on what I was going to do and I would not worry about my opponent. I'd heard Sena tell me things like: "Give them nothing, but take away everything from them." Or "First and foremost, always focus on you. You can't be concerned about what your opponent is bringing to the table." Or "Timidity allows doubt to creep in, which leads to improper form. A lot of people don't know anything—but if they act with boldness, even though they may be wrong, they will outperform others."

All the things that Christy, Sena and Royce had said to me during those months became like my mental control panel during my pre-fight.

Round Eight

THE FIGHT

Before my diagnosis, every so often, I'd pause while working the mitts and look up at Sena in the center of the ring to ask the crucial question. "If I was threatened, had to defend myself, or found myself in a dangerous situation, do you think I'd have it in me to *really* hit someone, touch my fist to another person's skin?" Taking a few seconds before resuming, he'd look away, chuckle and with careful thought respond, "Only if someone was going after your kids."

Coming from a not-so-safe home life, I had worked hard as a young adult to get my emotions in check and control an explosive and quick temper. When I found out about my cancer diagnosis, *It* now stood clearly before me—*It* being the universe and the dilemma I suddenly found myself in. I despised myself for feeling this, a primitive anger for wanting to bring about physical harm to *It*. I'd feel a disgusting taint of shame and the burden of failure for still holding onto this anger. Inside myself, I held contempt for the chaos and personal damage *It* represented, ready and eager to knock it down and beat up the circumstances I was in. The unfairness of the situation, and what it was taking away from me, made me want to invite some trouble—starting off by cursing *It* with the worst obscenities, provoking *It*, raising my fist and shouting at *It* and not caring who heard, showing my superiority and strength, physically fighting *It* in a serious beatdown, and keep pounding away until it couldn't speak another word to me. Maybe *It* would now understand *me* better. *It* had crossed my path and cut me off, was coming aggressively after me at the wrong time in my life, going after my deepest hopes, desires, and goals. Then, as I turned around and walked away from *It*, I'd take a deep breath and get back to the normalcy of my life and work to accomplish all my future goals.

I realized I was used to getting what I wanted, when I wanted it, and I was ready to revert to this comfortable situation where my schedule revolved around normalcy and not chemo treatments and surgeries. I felt I didn't deserve this. Sick and tired of behaving myself, trying so hard to lead a perfect life, doing all the right things—being a faithful and loyal wife for 25 years, working hard to secure the very best education for my sons, being the first mom to pull up for after-school pickup, staying healthy, preparing elaborate breakfasts for my family, and committing to a daily morning of meditation and prayer. I would suffer in passive torment, mask my anger with quiet resentment.

Rather than looking forward to advancing contracts with clients, my new future would be making conversations with strange doctors, nurses, and other chemo patients.

I'd curse the required daily progression logs that neatly tracked moods, and the blow-by-blow of what I ate and did throughout the day, like counting the number of times I chewed each bite at meals and personal details in the bathroom. In what felt like harassment, my nutritionist Virginia would gently nudge me to turn in my completed logs that had an inscription at the bottom:

Anything less than a loving thought is toxic. 1 logs was to add more balance to my life. I l the time to be nonsense paperwork, a sense waste of my time. My unending goal for ea two words: *feel joy.*

Then there were two things I craved all day and every day: muffins and chocolate chip cookies. Through late July, August and early September, I'd describe my feelings: "a constant headache; spacey with confusion, agitation that lasted all day, turning to a lot of worry, sadness, being afraid and angry." One Saturday morning, I clenched my jaw, feeling desperation as if I were struggling to stay afloat in this new life. I was in the parking lot at Royce's gym, trying not to unravel. But I did complain to Big Reggie, a not-so-big African-American man, a young gifted chef and dad to little Reggie. Royce would remind me that Reggie grew up in the Memphis projects, and because of his upbringing he knows no filter, which is a bonus to everyone he comes in contact with. Without giving any details of my cancer, I criticized the vegetables, burdock root and lotus root, and lamented all the things I could no longer eat or drink. He looked at me with steady eyes and a sweet smile and said something in a gentle voice that has stuck in my head forever: "Just be fascinated by your new lifestyle and all the new things you now get to eat." It felt like a sweet Mister Rogers moment, as if he was talking to a young child.

He was right. I readjusted my thinking and started to use this mantra every day. In mid-September, there'd be a sudden shift, like a change of the season, and I'd get a break. With my body

111

t resting on my forearm in a one-armed plank, I'd experience what Royce often said to me: "Kelly, it's only temporary discomfort, only temporary." My chronic headache and sadness changed to feeling joyful. By mid-September I wrote: *I feel inner peace and clarity and got rid of my headache.* A few days later I wrote, *I feel on top of my life.* I went from being headstrong and thrashing myself to trusting the process.

This new diet started making me feel more grounded and in control. I would start to hold on to my "new lifestyle" and the discipline it created to help me make it through. I found an unconventional way of managing fear through this diet and lifestyle. When I was feeling low, scared about what I was up against and frustrated by not being able to eat familiar foods, I heard Royce say, "it's a new lifestyle" and "no excuses, no complaints."

***

I felt the pull of contrary emotions in the early morning of September 24, but above all else, I was quietly pissed—to wake up at 4:30 a.m., be driven to a hospital, and start off my week waiting for hours. I have a low tolerance for waiting in a queue with uncertainty and insufficient information. I hated this place with its rows of connected seats and dull, humming fluorescent ceiling lights, off-white walls and wall-mounted TVs with cable news on. I was hungry and desperate for water and caffeine, and my skin was so tight and dry from being scrubbed with a special antibiotic soap that I felt like I was a desert dweller. I resisted looking around me, as if I'd be contaminated by making eye contact with anyone.

I reminded myself it's never too late to jump on a plane and run away. Sitting close to John, I looked up at him and felt weary, staying focused to hold on to all of my best. I was astonished to see the beautiful smile of my minister-lawyer friend Robin as she dashed into the waiting room a few minutes before my scheduled surgery, quickly directing us to hold her hands in prayer. In a call the night before, she had confirmed the time and place to pray for me. But it was a Monday, a workday for a single mom who managed an enormous career, and I was certain she wouldn't make it. I felt so loved at this moment. If she prayed for me, I was confident I would be okay. That this exact experience with Robin would be a constant thread over the next five months, I could never have imagined.

What happened next was like the ceremonial ringing of the bell. I heard "Susan Motley," the common 1970s name I changed in 5th grade to become Kelly. The calling of my first name set into motion a new clarity and the realization of all I had done to prepare for this moment. This was like that one morning when I walked into the gym to find Sena in his sparring equipment, was told to get into a ring that appeared to have shrunk, with me feeling overwhelmed and defeated in finding my breath.

I trudged forward with my head down. We were led to an elevator by a smiling, beautiful, 20-something African-American nurse. Her first mission would be to deposit John in a special family waiting area. My first reaction when John stepped off was

113

to scream out "NO" and lunge for him to stay with me. Saying goodbye to John felt like the ultimate version of going solo, inside the ring by yourself without your corner—or experiencing that common expression about how in death, no one will accompany you, you will exit life by yourself.

Since my diagnosis, I had hidden behind this man for protection and depended on him to know all the answers and to ask smart questions. As the chaotic and abrupt events began to unravel me, a change occurred in my marriage. My cancer would direct the course of our love and effortlessly push us to go deeper. John would become my cut man—the linchpin, whose job is to recognize when a fighter's health is at risk, to stop the bleeding in a 60-second timeframe, give physical support during the fight, deliver a calming message while making eye contact with the fighter, and be a decisive factor in the outcome of the match. In lockstep march with me, the fighter, he would help me get into fighting shape—preparing my mind and body for the abuse in the ring, cumulative blows, pain and major damage—just like a boxer receives in a full match with twelve rounds.

All my training would come into shiny focus when I walked into a temporary destination, a large staging-holding area of self-organized spaces with curtained boundaries for each patient headed to surgery. I ambled along behind the nurse, trying to be a detached observer, reminding myself again that it's never too late to run, feeling a tightness in my gut, paying close attention to hustling hospital personnel wearing green scrubs, noticing them at times glancing around at me and wondering why. I was led to my space, where I listened attentively to all kinds of instructions and responded to the same repetitive questions as if I was on a merry-go-round: Did I eat or drink fluids after midnight, are there any medications that I'm allergic to, and what's my birth date?

With a French accent, a sweet, attentive middle-aged nurse named Julia from the Democratic Republic of Congo would introduce herself and hand me a hospital gown, instructing me to get undressed and put all of my belongings into a large plastic bag. I stared at the plastic bag and made a mental note, telling myself that my double mastectomy surgery was probably nothing compared to escaping the violence and threatening times that my kind nurse went through to get to Nashville. Taking off my clothes, I thought back to her country's history and King Leopold II of Belgium's viciousness. Did I remember correctly that this king killed 10 million Africans, looted her country, amputated and mutilated the country's people, even children, as a means of control? Standing there naked, I worked hard to remember how to wear a gown that had only two options. I pulled off each shoe and sock, following Julia's instructions.

I wrestled with not giving myself over to cowardly thoughts. In a hospital gown, I firmly gripped my phone. I had secret plans to hold on to it. I had taught myself how to cling to order when there really isn't any, or when in a trapped, confined, cramped and enclosed situation where the air is insubstantial. I'd use trickery and deception, looking at what was most important to me, staring at it intensely to block out where I was and the people around me so that I could get into a flow. This worked well for me when sitting on a tarmac for hours in a turned-off plane or when trapped shoulder-to-shoulder in a suddenly broken-down monorail or stopped elevator. My photos and videos of my kids, of me working the mitts, recalling the songs I had trained to in the ring would keep me centered. Julia came and attached compression devices, squeezed onto my legs with an attached air pump. I asked her questions about the political situation in her former country after Mobutu's dictatorship. Later, my younger nurse and I would talk about Big Frieda, and I'd introduce her to a then up-and-coming independent musical artist, Lizzo. She would play for me the song "Rent" by Big Frieda, and I'd play her Lizzo songs. I'd scroll through my boxing training videos and photos of my sons on family vacations. I felt how the universe somehow gave me the two best nurses in the world.

I saw the back of my young polished plastic surgeon carrying a Prada briefcase passing my area. I had done my due diligence, interviewing half a dozen surgeons, and felt I had selected the very best to reconstruct my breasts. A few minutes later, he was mapping out the surgery with his black Sharpie, drawing circular patterns on my breasts to show the incision areas, this being part of the order, part of the process.

Into my curtained area a friendly, late-50s anesthesiologist introduced himself. He sat down next to me, looked down at the inside of my left elbow, smiled and told me, "Wow, I can see your veins from the moon." The site and sensation of injecting a needle into my veins triggered a deep sense of doom, as if I might lose consciousness. There was something foreboding about the needle entering my body, along with the sensation of possible excruciating pain. I have hated needles since I was a little girl. There would be my high-pitched screams, me flailing my arms about and being physically restrained by multiple adults when I got shots. As an adult, when it was time for my sons to get their shots at the pediatrician's office, I looked away from them, terrified for all of us.

Right then, my anesthesiologist made the announcement that he would break protocol. What he had just said was obviously preposterous to the nursing team: today, he'd be the one to start my IV. *I lucked out*, was my initial thought. Grateful, relieved to have the most qualified medical professional starting my IV, I was confident this was a good sign. I gazed to my right shoulder, then felt him fumbling. Thinking it was over, I looked up in the air to see my blood spraying out, pools on the floor, with him asking the nurses to clean up the blood.

Right before surgery, an unfamiliar nurse outside of my area would enthusiastically tell me that today was my lucky day, as if I'd be the patient in pre-op who just won a fabulous prize. She was excited about the drug I'd never heard of before, Dilaudid, and announced its street value.

The next thing I remember was waking up in a room looking at John. I had just made it through what seemed to be an inexplicable morning—a double mastectomy and having my breasts replaced with temporary, inflatable metal tissue expanders designed to stretch my skin and make room for future implants, with lymph nodes removed from under my right arm. Lymph nodes and tissue expanders; these were things I had never heard of before. In just a few weeks, there would be the next surgery. Into my upper left chest a silicone bubble would be implanted with a catheter attached that was threaded into a central vein—a port.

John was standing over me. I thought to myself, *he still loves me.*

Even with my chest bandaged, I suffered the greatest anguish from four long tubes inserted into my breast area, rib cage and armpits, with clunky plastic bulbs regularly filling up with blood and bodily fluid hanging, when they were not wound up, past my knees. The purpose of the surgical drains was to collect excess fluid in the area where the tumor had been, and the plastic bulbs on the ends created suction. They were painful—and psychologically, there was something about being horrifically stuck, with these tubes attached to my inner self, something I couldn't remove. I carried around these bags pinned to the waistline of my pants, crying, walking around my house and working. For weeks, I obsessed over desperately wanting to rip them out. Every second of every day, I had to restrain myself from screaming.

Even though it had only been a few days since my surgery and I was carrying these bags around the house, I had made up my mind I wasn't going to miss the photo op of my younger son's school dance with his date. My good friend and acupuncturist Dr. Xiao Mei Zhao warned me not to go. I tried to tuck the four bulbs full of blood into my baggy shirt and white jeans, with John driving all four of us to the school. From time to time, one or two of the bloody bulbs would randomly pop out. When I saw a group of parents on campus, one dad walked toward me, wrapped his arms tightly around me and squeezed me in the biggest, strongest hug of my life. Then he lifted me up off the ground for what seemed like eternity. A phenomenon like voltage spread across my being—a cracking boom of white light, a gigantic spark, possibly the most dangerous type of lightning, carrying 300 amps, had hit me. I heard what I thought was a huge explosion of my tissue expanders, like someone had punched me hard in the chest. My whole body froze up, and I was certain this would end with me being lifted off and then thrown to the ground. Pushing my tongue against the roof of my mouth, I held back my scream. The huge percussive force ended, and I landed back on my feet, lightheaded, trying to smile while breathing heavily, worried about the damage to my metal rounded boobs.

For weeks, I didn't have the guts to look at my own chest wounds; John would study them several times a day, really look at me. All the past trivial stuff we used to fight about—poof!— vanished. It was like someone hit the reset button on our relationship. When driving to appointments, we could have been on a first date, giddy, laughing, our fingers entwined in a tight grip, absorbed in each detail.

I had one month to get ready for chemotherapy (Herceptin and Taxol) with a start date of October 25. I'd go out of my mind on a one-hour shopping trip and buy expensive new clothes and shoes for a big client event in Chicago. I flew to Chicago with my tissue expanders all blown up, lined up a meeting with the editor and publisher of one of the biggest healthcare trade publications for an unknown client, and got terrific media coverage for the client.

***

Two days before I was to start chemo, while preparing myself for what I thought would be the worst, I was blindsided. I was at my computer, right in the middle of securing media coverage for an unknown healthcare technology CEO and his company. The afternoon phone call came out of the blue, at a tongue-twisting speed, with sing-song urgency.

It was my oncologist, and apparently, she was busy. I worked to decipher why she was calling me. She had already put the breast cancer plan in place. As I understood things, she was supposed to be my starting quarterback with all the cancer treatment plans in place, including scheduled surgery dates, a port in my chest, and the exact timing of 12 chemo treatments once a week.

We had just met with her a few weeks ago. At this appointment she had told John and me in a businesslike fashion that after *three* chemo treatments, the entirety of my hair *would* indeed fall out. She explained the future scenario of my hair loss and the other twenty or so side effects. This doctor bore a striking resemblance to Rosalie Mullins, the tightly wound, benevolent principal from the 2003 film *School of Rock*. With one leg neatly crossed over the other, she was telling me that losing my hair, eyelashes, and eyebrows was inevitable. Just like any expert calling a match, sometimes they get it right, but other times they get it wrong. (What she didn't know was that I was planning to be the odd woman out on this one.)

Now the relentless rhythm of her voice on my phone conveyed that she had other patients waiting and whatever was happening right now was taking too much time from her busy schedule. She'd string words together like: "We didn't get approval from your insurance company for the recommended treatment, and we need to proceed with more aggressive drugs three times as long, with more harmful and stronger side effects."

"Can you say it again?" I felt my whole being sliding out of my Marimekko pink poppy print chair and onto the hardwood floor. I was hearing the phrases *three times as long and stronger side effects* ringing like a bell in my head. I was becoming too tired to think.

I wasn't accustomed to typing these odd and now intensely personal words I'd never heard before: *the new treatment.* My immediate circumstances and the space around me were widening. I was feeling lethargic and incompetent at typing her bundled-up words, as though an irritated teacher was standing over my shoulder during a math test, with me running out of time. I was slowing her pace. I listened to her breathing that indicated she was losing her patience and would be done with me at any second.

Like being diagnosed with breast cancer, I never thought this could happen to me. I was smug on the topic of healthcare insurance, never seeing myself in the same pool as the millions of uninsured people I had read about. I worked to pull my heavy self out of this dreamlike state of disarray and return to the objective, professional self I had been just a few minutes ago. My skeptical instinct around sloppy business practices in healthcare kicked in. No way would I have an insurance company prescribing my treatment; that was a contradiction for a healthcare professional. Someone in her office was being sloppy or simply didn't want to spend additional time straightening out the situation with the insurance bureaucracy.

I said, "Surely we can work this out." The response: "There is nothing further my office can do."

My mind was blank. I no longer knew what to say. But I wasn't finished yet, nor was I going to let her hang up. I'd confront this problem. I told myself: *I make miraculous publicity things happen for people, sometimes by an easy conversation or simply typing a few words in an email.* This was too large a situation to just be complicit, even though I was finding it hard to find the strength to champion myself. I let her know my next steps: I would talk with my insurance company to get this matter resolved today and get everything cleared up.

"Oh, and who should I contact in your office once I get it resolved with our insurance company?" The turning point would be her next words, discouraging me from calling my insurance company. There would be nothing she or I could do to resolve the matter.

Right then I hoped for a different future, knowing this new treatment would damage me even more, take at least twice as much time away from my family, training, and running a business. What I really heard her say was: *I don't value your life, too much time would be wasted trying to convince the insurance company otherwise, so why bother?*

How could she not understand what this would cost me? I couldn't fathom that I was having this experience on a normal summer day. All of my choices were narrowed down to this. This felt perverse. I didn't have the strength to start looking around for a new oncologist. I had just let go of my cancer surgeon after feeling dismissed.

My voice buckled as I broke the news to John in consonants and vowels, trying to form words that sounded primitive. He got on the phone immediately with our insurance company and by the end of the day, he and I had coordinated a conference call with the oncologist's office administrator and an insurance representative. The case was run through the insurance system for a pre-approval to ensure there were no issues; we were given codes from the doctor's office for the original treatment. The insurance company communicated that all would be good and the oncologist's original treatment plan would be approved. Kelly would win this battle.

Round Nine

CHEMO

It would hide secretly beneath my skin. Only 1.5 cm in diameter. I had a bad feeling from day one when I learned about the port. As Royce might say, "I gave it energy." The idea of foreign materials implanted at the surface of my skin seemed not even for a moment like a good idea. My gut feeling was that my skin didn't seem thick enough for such an apparatus. But I cringed at the alternative: Walking around with bruises, raised bright red or pink puncture marks, scabs, scarring, and a discoloration running the length of the veins in my arm, as if I was shooting up. I'd need to dress like a junkie for the rest of my life, wearing long-sleeved shirts to hide the pock marks on my arms. Chronic injecting in the same spot over time would create collapsed veins and track marks and then I'd be in communion with *them*, searching desperately to find good veins for my weekly infusions.

I found that the theme around my conversations with doctors was that the port would be a breeze, risk-free. I'd be casually told that other than contact sports, I could swim and do anything and everything I wanted. All of this seemed like nonsense, too careless when talking about an implanted triangular silicone bubble beneath my skin, its location 3 cm below my left collarbone. Attached would be a thin, flexible tube that would sit in a large blood vessel leading to my heart. Maybe this device would be the one thing to pluck out my heart and leave me drowning in my blood.

My heart had never really captured my attention until now. I had neglected how this part pumps blood essential to carrying oxygen and nutrients to cells, organs and muscles to function, how it sustains and maintains me—physically, emotionally, giving me intention. My heart is the epicenter for my strength, determination, passion, and creative energy. The only thing that ever occurred to me when thinking about my heart was how it shuts down, the aftermath of how I abandon myself and cease the ability to feel kindness or tenderness toward myself.

I would have a rubber access site in the middle of the port where a needle would be perpendicularly pushed into my skin, into the device until it hits its bottom, with a small space between the needle and the skin line to prevent infiltration of fluid under the skin. I agonized about how my body would react to all these foreign materials implanted into it. But I obsessed about the durability of the situation, this object resting at the surface of my skin—that it might pop out as I was boxing, jumping rope and strength training. Going back and forth, I questioned whether I was being negative or overthinking a situation that millions of people agree to. This device would allow easy access for injecting fluid into my veins as part of my chemo treatment. I would avoid countless needle sticks and vein complications. When it came down to it, it would just be easy for me, easy for them, easier for my life, easier for theirs. No bruises. Simple for us all. Plus, I'd be told, I'd barely notice the lump in my skin and it would save the veins in my left arm, because I couldn't get blood from my right arm after the lymph nodes were removed. The reason was compelling; I understood its value but not its safety. (I was less well-informed about the critical word "sterile" and the con-tamination dangers of frequent access from the outside into the mechanism and the strict care required by my nurses.)

There was urgency for me to decide quickly for the upcoming chemo treatments. Perfectionism was at play when trying to make the best decision here. "What's the worst that could hap-pen?" I asked myself, and I ultimately agreed to have a port placed under my skin. I was cut at the base of my neck and then a second cut on my chest, under my collarbone, where a catheter was tunneled under my skin from the second cut back to the first to create a path from the port to the access site on my neck, threaded into a vein. With a blunt dissector, my new doctor cre-ated a 2-cm pocket for the port underneath it. She'd close all of this with sutures and skin glue.

Things kicked off early that day with the strangeness of the here and now. Ambushes are based on information gathering, a deli-cate approach—the purpose being to strike fear in hearts, emerg-ing from obscurity to deliver a sudden punch.

Chemo is a horrible concept that happens to other people, I thought. Something that originated from the mustard gas warfare of World War I would be pumped into my body today. I'd be forever connected to the former WWII scientists who discovered that chemical agents could destroy or control the growth of cancer cells. The hypothesis was that if mustard gas could slow down the growth of white blood cells, it could also destroy cancerous ones.

It felt like madness to be linked to a deceased, Harvard-educated botanist and the highly poisonous 25-foot Pacific yew tree. Humans have used yew since the dawn of history for making poisonous weapons and bows, and the Greeks and Romans believed it had a mythological association with death. A few years before I was born, there were collections of bark, stem and fruit samples from the yew tree by a botanist working for an arm of the USDA in Washington State as part of the government's approach toward plant exploration for medicinal properties. From this a natural compound, paclitaxel, would be created to destroy cancer cells. It would become the cancer drug Taxol, killing cancer cells in ways scientists had not previously imagined.

We endured the check-ins, long waits, checking my blood count, then we were off to the infusion area for pre-meds, which are given 30 to 60 minutes before the chemo to reduce nausea and allergic reactions. We were moved into a large, free-standing rectangular room filled with rows of buttery leather recliners called clinical infusion chairs, each chair with its own IV pole. There was a steady stream of young African-American women briskly walking from behind a counter for the administration of dangerous, strong, toxic potions. Oncologists walked down a spacious polished corridor, avoiding eye contact with the reclining crowd in the room, speaking to us only in their designated private offices.

"Holy shit" was my feeling. I'd never seen this as my reality. I hated *It* even more now, this cancer and the situation, for the wickedness and poor timing in wounding each person's life—the man or woman who, in my eyes, was either too young, too feeble and frail, had worked too hard, had gone through this before, hadn't had the chance to have kids, or would never know what it's like to be married.

Trudging, almost stumbling, in my new Alexander Wang boots, I looked around and found no best option on where to sit for getting my infusion. I lay back and waited, completely exposed. I was hooked up to my own IV pole with a needle in my port dripping saline solution. I still held on to the illusion of having the upper hand and control of my universe. After an hour and a half, we realized a sudden change in the sequence—not a soul was around to administer my pre-meds or a steroid for nausea, and no one had ordered the chemotherapy. We waited for another hour and a half.

Then suddenly a thunderous rush of feet came toward us. There was confusion, misunderstanding, maybe deception. A band of nurses and a young insurance administrator converged around us. The two of us would take on the strength of many, as though we were villagers on a tortuous road cornered in a surprise attack and now intimidated. There was a mass of paperwork and we heard familiar words from a few days ago that were not supposed to be relevant. Like a hated song stuck in my head, the surprise billing issue over my treatment plan resurfaced. In a chorus, the nurses were saying that my treatment would not be covered by our insurance. It felt like an interrogation, and I wanted to leave.

I failed to grasp what they were saying about a new course of treatments. I felt like I was starting to float away. We heard that a much longer period of time for chemo would be needed: three times the length would be their recommendation. We didn't expect this. They pushed paperwork and pens in front of us, saying that if we went with the original treatment plan, we'd need to sign forms accepting responsibility for each $40,000 treatment. I felt an overwhelming sense of chaos as I looked up at the IV pole attached to me. Wanting to vanish, I felt pinned there by thin plastic tubes that could have been chains or ropes. If there had been an opportunity to scoot out of the recliner, crawl out of this place and tiptoe out, I would have seized it, but I couldn't find an easy route to maneuver.

The doctor's recommended twelve weeks of chemo treatments of Taxol and Herceptin now seemed too good to be true. I heard my doctor's words from a few days ago, "three times as long with much more aggressive side effects," and slip in and out of an imaginary world. But in reality, John and I had worked out this financial matter with my insurance company, the doctor, and her office. Hadn't we just met with the doctor and heard agreement about the regular treatment?

But we would now be deceived. The nurses and administrator had concerns about the insurance company paying the doctor for her recommended treatment plan of targeted therapy for HER2-Positive breast cancer by using Herceptin and Taxol. I heard John say with no hesitation, "I'm not going to risk my wife's life with a more devastating treatment. I will sign the form." These words were spoken by a sensible man whose whole being is driven by the safety of his family.

So onward we went as we took control. My heart raced as the needle went into the port in my left chest area. I'd be in a desperate situation and say I was sorry. How does anyone prepare to meet a supreme decree, a hideous diabolic phantom that feels like Beelzebub in disguise? Chemo could be like the description in the Second Book of Samuel, an "angel who was working destruction among the people." By just trying to heal, I'd be inviting a dark, shadowy creature into my human soul. It would be sudden. There'd be a deliberate pattern every week after my treatment. You watch yourself slowly slip away. It's like that one relationship in your life where the other person has a way of taking from you or doing something that hurts you, while maintaining that it was *all* for your own good.

I'd been getting myself ready for a sneaky, deliberate opponent that would start off subtly, deliberately damaging me in my first encounter when I'd be given just enough to suspect something wasn't right. But I started to understand that I will be the one constantly hurt—wounded, entwined by these mighty hands. I would strive to constantly make adjustments so as not to lose. I'd take a punch so hard that the tips of my toes and fingers would be cold, burn and tingle with pain, years later, maybe for eternity. Whatever this thing was, it struck me dumb. As if inhaling combustion fumes, I endured a colorless gas, smog, like inhaling too much incense from a church service, fogging up my head.

Nothing would be crystal clear and I'd have memory slips that caused me panic. At the grocery store checkout, I forgot my own PIN number, based on the most important day of my life. The name of the man, Richard, who once held my mitts for me during Jeet Kune Do workouts would now escape me. I'd doze, bored to tears listening to a nurse give me instructions, and fall asleep a few inches from her face. I'd be baffled by my inability to focus, a loss of concentration that felt like a cousin to dementia. A day spent multi-tasking would no longer exist for me. Royce and Sena would have to give me more frequent, repeated instructions on what they wanted me to do next in my training.

I fought for my existence after each round of chemo by opting for the YMCA rather than bed. Each week John and I had a ritual of going from chemo to the gym, getting on an elliptical for an hour and throwing punches with five-pound weights. I treated the situation as if I was drinking too much alcohol and I created my own personal belief that exercise would help metabolize all the poisons more quickly. During this time, I resembled a frail old woman at the downtown Y, cautiously, barely tapping the speedbag, concentrating hard to form circles with my wrists.

***

A month after my surgery in October, I sent a note to Royce asking if I could stretch in the corner of the gym. The smallest of movements, extending my legs and bending forward, now seemed absurd. Royce looked at me in disbelief after a month of not seeing me at the gym. Using the *can't* word is forbidden with Royce, but even the smallest of movements seemed damaging to my body. Before leaving the gym, I expressed my interest in training with him three days a week to start regaining my strength. Along with strength training, I got to hit the mitts with Royce.

A few days after he won his fight in December, I started back training with Sena. We worked consistently three early mornings a week, even the day before and after Christmas, the two of us shuffling around to different gyms in Nashville. The day I started back with Sena, I went directly from a chemo treatment to meeting him at the Y. I pulled my car into the street parking lot, fatigued, unable to move, sitting in my car, with what felt like an odorless gas in my head, heart and organs. I did something that was unthinkable before my diagnosis. Laying back my car seat in downtown Nashville, I shut my eyes and took a nap. And when I woke up, it took every force in my being to step out of the car to meet Sena. For inspiration, I reflected back on what Royce said about keeping a strong mindset: "Let the mind override the body, when the body gets tired."

After this workout, I walked away with a new understanding about the power of this mitt training, helping me to see what I was going through was less of a battle. I would see it as a game, with a new clearness, and it seemed to depollute my mind and body from all the toxins. Pushing myself physically with this workout helped me to recover from the treatments.

During this period, I'd suddenly awaken each night, visited by the sight of my death. There would be a frantic plea to be spared. A black, malevolent winged creature of darkness sitting at my bedside would come to torment me, to remind me I was no longer fierce, telling me to surrender. It felt like a rape—dwelling in me, reigning over me, wreaking havoc, dancing over me, scorching me, wrapping me up and drinking my breath. Warfare was going on inside my body with a transparent, heavy, evil shadow killing off my spirit. I woke in the middle of the night terrified of this obscene thing that was both in me and hovering on top of me, trying to steal me. I craved life.

My only refuge was to see the wrinkled, veined, willful, strong hands of my maternal 104-year-old great-grandmother sweeping down over my body for protection, saying, "That's enough." She who cared for me with her tireless hands that held me in her lap, even as an adult in my 20s. I recalled how she put her one fingertip to her mouth when dealing cards, how she used her fingers to tap an inch-long ash from her cigarette. Hands to sew, to strip a branch from a tree to make a switch when I disobeyed, to garden, rake, pick up leaves, iron, fold clothes, push a grocery cart with me in it, cook, and brush her long gray hair that went to her ankles, then wind it up on her head with Victorian hairpins. Terrified, I hoped summoning her would somehow make this black angel miraculously go away, and then I'd tightly curl up next to John to bury my face firmly into his back.

***

I was told no form of nutrition or supplement would help raise my white blood cell count (WBC). I had an inexplicable compulsion to solve this problem. I spent hours researching and casually slipped in a question at every touchpoint I had with a healthcare professional. I hit the same dead end every time. I believed deep down that my nutritionist Virginia's recommended shots of liquid chlorophyll and liquid plant iron sucked through a straw in the back of my mouth, turning my teeth black, were helping me. In silence, I questioned why no one had an answer to my obsession.

Most of my life, I had panicked at numbers, but now numbers like 3.8 would start to be my new language. Just like Pythagoras said, "Numbers rule the universe." Everything was organized around this one number at the intersection of everything I did. Numbers would be my sign that told me that my body could no longer protect itself or was at a higher risk of infection. I'd search for the frequency of number patterns telling me how the chemo was affecting me. Overnight the numbers would plummet, and I'd sink into discouragement. Throughout my chemo treatment I was consumed, fretting with this one detail that told me if I was below normal and vulnerable. It also would be my dashboard, indicating whether I'd have to prolong this horror of chemo, pushing treatments out to what felt like a shrinking future.

After my desperate pleas to lift my WBC numbers, Virginia told me, "Go ahead and increase dulse seaweed. Use it in your food to cook with or as a condiment. You can get dulse flakes or toast the dulse and crumble it over your food. Add more greens and beets to your program." I was spot-on in following her every detail. I'd consume the meat of umeboshi plums and perform daily meditations where I willed my numbers to go up. Dr. Zhao recommended 20 goji berries a day. My numbers once gloriously skyrocketed, and I was validated that going on a restful trip to the beach had been the reason. During week nine of chemo, my white blood cell count got so low, my new doctor wanted to push back my weekly chemo treatments. I wasn't going to let this happen. I needed to get through these twelve weeks of chemo and move on with my life. I'd asked her at each appointment the same nagging question about how to raise my WBC count.

This day, I calmly asked her again. She looked at me as though she was giving me the answers to a test, and leaned forward. My persistence paid off. I'd find the secret to raising my white blood cell count. This was something easy for me to do: high cardio activity right before my blood draws. Rather than taking the escalator as I went in for chemo, I climbed the long set of stairs 20 times up and down until my name was called out in the converted shopping mall lobby. I then went into the private office of a nurse whose space resembled a vortex shop out of Sedona, with peacock feathers, unicorns on the wall inscribed with "Believe in Magic," and stickers of forest animals for a baby's nursery with the phrase "Hope is the anchor of the soul." I put on some AC/DC, jumped rope, and did an intense 80s-style form of aerobics for a good five minutes before the blood draw.

Work meant something altogether different to me during chemo. Chemo helped me to evolve my work, forced me for the first time to have a greater sense of balance with my business, gave me greater confidence by testing my mental faculties, and became a diversion from the insanity of cancer. At first, it seemed incomprehensible that I could maintain the mental abilities to work.

Understanding chemo's side effects, I was fairly certain I would become dumb, no longer able to write and distribute media releases, unable to convince reporters and editors to cover clients for media coverage, manage weekly calls with a CEO, or continue to build brands.

My biggest fear was being worthless. Not having a career devalued me. I felt immense pride once a year when sitting down with my accountant. His face would light up, he'd hug me and praise me for being a female lioness who takes down large prey for the family. So much of my personal identity for my adult life was tied up in my profession. I had a need to feel valued and worthwhile, and I liked attention and impressing others with my PR skills. First and foremost, I was Will and Alex's mom and John's wife. But my identity anchor also was tied up in the accomplishments I could get for my clients and in exceeding expectations.

I couldn't understand initially what the diagnosis meant for my business and income. Or more importantly, who I would be or who I would now become. I felt the rapid shrinking of my professional world and sense of self. To be associated with cancer would be terrible for my business. Any vulnerabilities I ever showed in the workplace had backfired. In the real world, there was very little talk, ever, about my personal life. I understood that my work is about getting results. Everything was diminishing as I had a feeling of hopelessness: what would this do to my professional world and my newly executed plan to grow my business?

Clients weighed me, a solo practitioner, against PR agencies and teams of professionals. Ironically, two months before my diagnosis, I was driving through Kentucky when a prospective client called to ask me a never-before-posed question that I considered preposterous, even hysterical. I was spellbound, tongue-tied, and needed to pull my car to the side of the road. The COO asked, "We are more interested in hiring you, but we are concerned: what if something happens to you?" In complete disbelief, I'd later share this implausible scenario with John, and we would just laugh. I knew my own party line: *All the women in my family live into their hundreds.*

A friend showed me how to leverage work to get through the chemo treatments. With optimism and in the coolest way, my Meharry doctor friend Regina said to me, "You know, Kelly, some women work through breast cancer as a distraction. It's done all the time. Women work through this while also introducing it as a strategy to help move forward." This was coming from the same woman who had smiled and encouraged me to stay unflappable a year before when I was flailing, frustrated by a CEO's last-second wait to sign our contract. (Eventually I got the contract signed.)

To find new strength for taking on cancer, I got the same recommendation from all of my doctors and my nutritionist Virginia: get rid of any stressors in my life. I knew right away what this meant. *Yes,* I now told myself, *this is the time for me to dump my one messy client who led me to boxing—the one who brought negative energy to me, required huge amounts of my time and required defensive strategies. The one who seemed to know how to exploit my weaknesses and overrun my boundaries.* I'd honor the two-month notice in my contract and tell them: "I am restructuring my business, moving to a different service model, and thank you for this terrific opportunity." This one decision helped me to rethink. I would be working only with people who would be good for my business during this period of my life.

Round Ten

HAIR

"Oh, Kelly, MY clients don't lose their hair," Virginia said, leaning into me emphatically, eyeball to eyeball across her desk. That was all I needed to hear. Losing my hair would be classified as a radical concept with no further discussion. I trusted Virginia's track record of saving hundreds of lives, even her own, proving bigwig doctors wrong when they insisted her food treatment might have been black magic. Her response gave me the emphatic belief that I was still in charge of my world, with or without breast cancer— and no, I certainly would not lose my hair.

However, seven months after completing my chemo treatments, I was sitting in my sunlit music room talking on the phone with my friend Sarah about my hair regrowth. Formerly stick-straight and 25 inches long, it was now about two inches long on top and was coarse yet kinky, wavy, definitely fluffy and, in some places, curly. It was growing, but at different rates at different places on my head. The sides were experiencing fast growth, but the left side was growing back more quickly than the right. The front and crown seemed more stagnant. I was struggling with styling it and how to shape it. The dialogue was like two old men talking about grass or crops and all the factors that influence their growth. All the suffering and anxieties around my hair loss vanished with the smallest bit of new hair resurfacing, giving me a new reassurance and gratitude, causing me to quit obsessing about what was missing from my life.

I moved on to my obsession about my low white blood cell count. I shared with Sarah that I had my blood taken for the first time since my breast reconstruction surgery five months earlier, and my blood and immune cells were not rebounding. In our conversation, I slid in something that Virginia had told me a few months ago: the accumulation of multiple rounds of chemo— the remnants of drugs—stays in your body for up to *seven years* after treatment, with lingering side effects. *Seven years.* Virginia had shared this warning with me so that I would keep taking my bulk of daily supplements. In my conversation with Sarah, I then paused and said, "Well, who knows if this is true or not."

Sarah responded laughingly in her always soft, smooth voice, "Oh right… is this the same woman who said, 'Kelly, MY clients don't *lose* their hair'? Did you turn to her later and point to your head and say, 'What about this, bitch?!'"

Sarah seemed like the only person on the planet (including me) who really comprehended the seriousness of my situation. She called every week and wanted meticulous updates on my health, taking notes, doing follow-up research, sending her investigative findings and asking me in her messages after surgeries: "Are they giving you enough pain killer?" At one point, she even booked a last-minute flight during a Northeastern snowstorm to come from Boston to Nashville to sit by my side at the hospital.

You'd be hard-pressed to find another living soul on this planet like my friend Sarah. I was coming home from a preppy Virginia school at 16 for the summer and, when I first met her, I imagined her introducing herself and saying, "Hi, I'm Sunshine." Wearing only hippie skirts and flowing dresses, ginger-haired and freckled, Sarah always looked more like a Rocky Mountain goddess with grace, kindness, and sensibility than a mortal woman. She was a few years older, with an overabundance of hip-length, blazing red, wavy hair, and she grew up on a ranch in Colorado riding horses with hardy, rugged cowboys. As a free-spirited 18-year-old, she was perfectly comfortable strolling around naked in the California scene at the Esalen Institute. I remember seeing a picture of her in long braids in the mountains of West Virginia, where she created a Vietnam veterans' retreat with her much older millionaire boyfriend. In college she started a profitable catering business for thoroughbred racing events. She knew the world and had backpacked across Europe several times. For a few years, she was a steady presence in L.A.'s poorest and most dangerous neighborhoods, working with gangs, sex workers, the homeless, transgender people and porn actors on how to prevent sexually transmitted diseases. The way she lived her life would one day make a headline story in *The New York Times* with her featured foster dog Lucie. Lucie was later described in her obituary as "a mangy, emaciated, Lyme-afflicted dog with bad bowels."

Sarah's way of seeing injustice in the world was always presented with the most upright principles. Seeing a dog locked in an SUV with its windows tightly sealed on a hot summer day, she would write a surprisingly friendly note to leave on the windshield: "Hello Friend! Leaving your dog in your car on a hot day like today with the windows up is risky, as he could become seriously ill." She fled a 20-year marriage, whacking off her hair, and never looked back.

Sarah helped me to discover unwavering confidence that, as a 16-year-old kid with a laminated ID, I could make it into a bar. At times we even walked in together with Sarah's face on two driver's licenses, with me using her out-of-state West Virginia ID. I felt I could go anywhere, without any questioning, and present her old license, make easy eye contact with the bouncer and make it inside. Never getting busted, stopped, or refused entry at a club's door, never getting her identification confiscated. We spent our summers dancing at bars. Five years after John and I started dating, she flew from L.A. to Kentucky to single-handedly cater a Martha Stewart-type wedding reception for John and me—free of charge.

Sarah's hair loss comment was a reminder of the vital message I had clung to every second of each day, one that I vehemently reiterated to myself and smugly declared to nurses, friends, and family. I had said it in the most logical, focused way: "Oh, my nutritionist told me I would not be losing my hair." People just nodded, or there would be a paused silence on the other end of the phone, as if *I* believed in imaginary things. I'd hoodwink chemo and its ability to make me go bald, because of my superior knowledge of this macrobiotic lifestyle. I'd follow the *I won't lose my hair script* and execute it with confidence.

Even when asking Virginia the hair question, I was petrified to bring up the subject, knowing at the time I was going against Royce's principles by asking her "what if" questions and introducing bad energy into the universe. I was being that fighter who shows doubt before stepping into the ring. But it was a reasonable question that couldn't be dismissed. At my first appointment, my then-oncologist told John and me in a businesslike fashion that after *three* chemo treatments, my hair *would* indeed fall out. She was seated in front of me with one leg neatly crossed over the other, telling me that losing my hair was inevitable. What she didn't know was that I'd be the misfit, the exception—all because of my eating.

Hair loss is the most visible sign of chemotherapy, but I'd miraculously make it through three, four, five chemo treatments with my long hair still intact. I knew the drugs were taking a devastating toll on my insides because of my low white blood cell count each week and the sores in my mouth. But, on the outside, I appeared physically fit, had not gained any weight, or lost my hair.

Some might think I was delusional or overly optimistic, that my fantastical thinking didn't match the real-world situation. Maybe I was holding on to a belief system that was no longer serving me. My diet became my way of embracing the madness. Feeling this certainty about not losing my hair gave me a level of comfort, a sense of order. Looking at the facts, I knew that life was unpredictable and there were inexplicable things happening to me, but keeping my hair didn't seem so far-fetched. And by God, it would be so!

On November 16, 2018, in an unmanageable way, my world was tipped on its side. I remember everything quite well as if I were the type of eyewitness that investigators would hope to find: that person whom others depend on for accurate and detailed recall. I remember the exact day, time, place, and vivid details. John was leaving our home that Friday for noon strength training with Royce. He had a routine of yelling goodbye to me on his way to the front door. He was loading his black gym bag into the back of his black SUV, which was parallel-parked on the street in front of our home.

There was a special excitement that day. Our older son, Will, would be coming home that evening for Thanksgiving break from Kenyon College. His college baseball coach described my son as "the most even-keel person you will meet in your life, hardworking, smart, and makes good decisions. Responsible, reliable, always professional." His summary of Will was: "He simply does exactly what he is supposed to do." I saw this in him, while I was raising him, in watching him attack the strike zone, and in the ways he supported me through cancer.

He brought this same steady confidence to me when he picked up his phone the minute I'd call him. I'd get more nurses interested in checking on me with Will sitting at my side during chemo infusions while he was on holiday breaks from school. His text message the night before my double mastectomy was about healing powers and how he was praying for me. With what I was up against, I wish I could have fast-forwarded and caught a glimpse of the future, after my final chemo treatment, when I'd see the best-pitched game of his college career—pitching the entire game, giving up two runs on two hits, winning 3-2. He coolly walked off the mound, approached and hugged me, and handed me the game-winning ball. I stared down at the ball in my hand and felt like a warrior.

I was styling my hair with a wooden paddle brush. We'd be picking Will up at the airport that evening, then leaving for a special family trip to Miami. I was looking down at the ugly 1980s plain cream linoleum floor with swirls of beige that I had wanted to replace. (It seemed remarkable that my darkest hour would be forever connected to this drab, worn-out floor covering.) I was away in my thoughts when I started to blow out my hair—then I was frozen by seeing the large, thick clumps of bronze, caramel-highlighted, long hair forming what could have been a shag carpet at my feet.

I turned off the blow dryer and let it drop into the empty old sink with a constant drip that no plumber in Nashville could ever fix. I now felt beyond human help. I had been quietly tidying up the single fallen hairs around me for the past month, on my pillows, off my shoulders and in the sink, as if this were normal.

I was tied to this desperate realization that I wasn't in charge. I *was* going bald, while trying to make sense of how I lost sight of so many good intentions. My real self had to cease pretending.

I thought back to the miso soup I now loathed but ate with fake enthusiasm for breakfast. I recalled how miso helped to heal Japanese monks after Hiroshima and thought its medicinal powers would help me, too. I would no longer have the stomach for eating a three-year fermented barley miso paste with Japanese sea vegetables. I was Virginia's model client, the high school goody-two-shoes valedictorian of eating clean and adopting a new lifestyle—just so this very thing would not happen. While most of my life I had felt like a troublemaker, skirting the rules and struggling with following directions, I had become the expert on following Virginia's instructions. If Virginia had said to lick the white lines on a paved road in a remote Tennessee county, I would have done it to save my hair. If she had told me to do this at a specific time of the day or week, I would have planned my schedule around it.

I now felt a weightlessness as if I were floating. The space between losing my hair and walking to the front door could have been a dream. I panicked at the idea of experiencing this paralysis alone. But I knew regimen and order were themes that permeated my husband's life story, and I would cause disruption to his time-table. I was introducing chaos into his sense of order. I found myself standing hunched over outside the front door, desperate for his help. I went mute on our front porch trying to call his name as he went to the car, opened the driver's side door and got in. I was praying that he would see me and not drive off. I tried to speak, yell, but could only use my breath without vocal cords to softly murmur, "John, John, John." I was winded like a winning sprinter interviewed on TV after a race, unable to catch a breath. I managed to wave and get his attention. He could have thought it was inconsequential. That I was waving him down as a reminder to pick up a needed ingredient for a recipe. But he got out of his car.

I'd never been so desperate in my life for help. My hair was clearly falling out. But it was more about the need to confess that I didn't have the power I thought I had. With all of what I was doing, I was failing. In a small voice, I whispered, "Hey, can you come here?"

Then I experienced something holy. Something sacred. Several life themes—power, truth, love—all intersected. If ever there was a cry of the human heart, this was it: expressing my own human frailty, a cracking of the illusion of being in control of my life while simultaneously experiencing the enveloping, perfect, agape love flowing perfectly from John to my soul.

He said in an easygoing tone, "What's up?" Bent over, I struggled to explain to my husband, in a faint voice, "I'm losing my hair." As if John had just read a how-to guide for talking with people in desperate situations, he listened intently, was logical and careful, understanding the value of using simple, precise words, achieving a perfect cadence. His tone was even and gentle. His next steps were simple, prescriptive: "OK, this is what we are going to do," he said, as he cradled my head in his hands. He then said slowly, "We are just going to stop brushing and washing our hair."

I stared back at my husband in rapture. All of a sudden there was power to step away and reset myself. He defused my desperation and changed the subject at the same time. I found temporary peace and understanding. My semblance of order had been temporarily restored. John offered to me a new framework, a playbook. I started to breathe, stood up straight and felt back on track. I had an advantage over this breast cancer. All I had to do was to stop brushing and washing my hair.

John looked magically different all of a sudden. I had a new realization: John *is* clever. Yes, it had escaped me just how incredibly smart my husband is—until this desperate, hopeless moment. Our eyes met. I loved him for his response. I now remembered that this *is* one of the reasons I married him. Standing before him now, I realized it had been worth the wait for him when he went off to France for almost a year before we got engaged. The compilation of an insane 150 credit hours of undergraduate college classes had just paid off. The man who took the highest level of math classes possible in college—Physics Student of the Year, four graduate semesters of Latin, securing three university degrees, plus almost a *Matrice* degree from a French university— had suddenly shared with me the tips for how to step away from this desperate situation.

With this "hands-off approach" of no washing or styling hair, I had a new looseness to life. The messy hippie hair would be just fine. My hair went from smooth to having its own wild, free, disheveled personality. I rationalized that shampoo was a clever commercialized campaign and no longer for me. The incident in the bathroom now seemed like a long time ago. On the flight to Miami a few days later with my family, I took photos of our sons and I was so happy, all of us together as a family, just the four of us, going to a place with good energy, and I wanted nothing more than to sit together on the beach.

But I noticed, when disembarking the plane, a new problem, one grown organically—that my uncombed hair had started forming a hard, impenetrable, matted mass of tangles on the back of my head. The weight of the entangled hair made me realize that what I was experiencing was altogether a different situation. I reassured myself, knowing my prized attribute is adaptability, telling myself, *you've got this.*

I'd need to create a new plan for dealing with this. I imagined therapeutic properties of sea water. I justified that once I got to the beach, I'd swim in the ocean and the sea water's nutrients and minerals would reverse my hair's tight tangles and knots that were quickly becoming one large lock. I'd imagine myself running straight into the ocean, my arms out, and diving into a wave. Ten seconds later, I'd come up for air and my fine hair strands would be disentangled, flowing in the water around me. Perhaps the ocean would help with the thinning issue as well, I surmised. This would be the beginning of multiple improvisational plans to keep from becoming hairless at age 51.

What I would discover after plunging my head into the ocean was that my hair would become more knotted, parched, and brittle, with the long hairs adhering together even tighter. Extras—pieces of marine algae, ugly thickish seaweed with tiny fragments of seashells—would be woven in, seemingly impossible to ever comb out. My next plan would be around headgear. I thought about Dwight Yoakum, appearing to have long hair, but in reality, having just strands of hair around a bald patch. His broad-brimmed hat perfectly hid his baldness. For the next few days, I built my hairstyle around a black Kenyon College baseball cap. I simply tucked my one massive lock up into my baseball cap, which looked as if I were tucking my long beach hair pony tail into it. I smiled and coordinated the cap with my outfits, and it served me well for sitting on the beach and going out in Miami. But I knew this look could only last so long. Plus, it was painful to sleep on this thick cable.

I leaned into my efficient Google searching skills. While few things in life come effortlessly to me, I have developed a keen proficiency, through my PR work, at finding just about anybody's contact information and reaching out to them. I thought getting the answer to detangling my hair would be a breeze. The night before leaving Miami, I searched phrases like "how to detangle severely matted hair," but reached an impasse.

My next plan involved saturating my head with a bottle of conditioner and relying on John's helping hands. That night in our hotel room, John cradled me in his arms, taking his time and gently trying to unravel obstinate knots with his fingers, breaking apart big clumps of matted hair, separating strands by pulling, pinching and untwisting. Nothing broke apart in this time-consuming endeavor while we watched family movies. After several hours, John, who could figure out anything, gave up.

In photos of me from Miami, my eyes are looking up and they show that I was grateful to be alive. But they reveal that I had been through something big, while surrounded by the physical and mental strength of my husband and two sons. You could see how the chemo was taking its toll on my skin and prematurely aging me. In every picture, I had shielded myself behind John, using him as a protective barrier against what I felt was a threat. I had positioned him to cover the vulnerable parts of me with just my head stuck out to the side of my family.

As we were leaving Miami, I awkwardly asked John if he would call Kyle before we boarded our flight back to Nashville. Kyle just so happened to be a pragmatic stylist, brought up in Grand Rapids, Michigan—he came from the same hometown as Floyd Mayweather Jr., considered to be one of the greatest pound-for-pound fighters. Kyle was born into a large Catholic family of blue-collar auto workers. As a young man, he had plunged himself into Catholicism and chosen the monastic life for a brief period in search of truth. He would touch my head like it was a sacramental act. For Kyle, touching another person's hair was an expression of trust. His reputation was based on his celebrity A-list clients, including one of the most famous actresses in the world. Surely, he had the skills to remedy this unusual situation.

A few minutes later, I watched John walk away from me and talk on his phone in a corner of the airport. First, I became consumed with the question, *What will happen to me if I can't get in to see Kyle?* It was a Saturday, the busiest day of the week for a stylist. And there was no Plan B in my mind. The explanation I would have to offer Kyle seemed far-fetched. There were no regular words for this. How would I rationally explain what had become of my hair to Kyle?

John is a smart negotiator, effortless, risk intolerant, and graceful in talking with people, and he knows how to get creative. Most importantly, he has a low-key style, and people genuinely like him. His smooth gait, as he approached me, communicated that he had secured a major business deal. "Be at the salon at 4:30 p.m."

At 4:28 p.m. on Saturday, November 24, 2018, I discreetly slid through the front door of Kyle's new salon, named after his party hostess grandmother, Bea Rose. I was apprehensive, timid, and giving myself a pep talk. But the appointment time itself said things might not be right. No woman gets her hair done this late on a Saturday in Nashville. On Saturdays, the busiest day of the week, salons close in the afternoon. I seated myself on the Hollywood Regency-style velour blue sofa that represented Bea Rose's infamous sofa in Detroit—the one that she literally took a saw to so that her husband would buy her a new, larger one for her weekend parties. I held a steady gaze at the floor, fixed on blending in with the surroundings, acting natural and going with the flow. I tried not to look up, avoiding eye contact. Like someone with a smiling face and a clenched fist, I presented a combination of signals that contradicted each other. Trying to appear confident but sliding off the couch, I was thinking long and hard about possible speaking points with Kyle. Just like the sacrament of confession, it would require preparation. I told myself I had this. I sat there and checked off my life milestones, obstacles I had overcome and positive life lessons that had helped me to navigate uncomfortable situations. I was the expert at pushing myself outside my comfort zone and doing things that, for some people, might seem terrifying. I told myself it was all good.

A man more naturally beautiful than the most beautiful of women approached me. I greeted Andrew, co-owner of Bea Rose and Kyle's husband, a man more expert at make-up than anyone I'd ever met. He was formerly known by the drag persona Angel Electra. I then took off my baseball cap. His face showed a mixture of intense fascination and horror. His expression showed me that what was underneath my cap was a catastrophe. I stammered, my voice searching for the missing words: "Oh, this, well, …This crazy thing happened to me in Miami."

Andrew sat down next to me, casually showing photo after photo of Kyle's most famous celebrity client. This was a calculated preparation for helping me put together a disaster recovery plan. A master artist, a great explainer of the fabric of reality, he subtly pointed out that something strange was going on—if only I would stop and look. A world was constructed in front of me that I had never analyzed. Maybe it was intentional blindness or my brain glossing over details. The images he showed me were of Kyle's celebrity client wearing wigs at the Golden Globes or in film roles. His gentle lesson was that wearing a wig is a common thing today. *Yes, it is a wig, but no one needs to know*, was his message. A best-kept secret. Women wear them for styling convenience, changing up a look, or feeling creative. I was going through something big in my life—so why not experiment with my hair? I started to weigh how I value my privacy and the normalcy of a wig. It would make me feel safe and be a good option.

When Kyle was ready to see me, he had already worked a full day cutting, coloring and blowing out the hair of at least fifteen clients, but he didn't let on that he was tired. I followed him back to his chair, the two of us alone together in an empty salon surrounded by ten stylists' chairs. Confession around human failure is an ancient practice. I was the guilt-burdened person who had come up short, having a real fear of telling a priest my sins and being judged. I tried for the exact words. I started reviewing what had seemed like, at the time, rational steps, and searched for words for how I earnestly approached my hair. But the hopeless facts remained. I said, "Well, I just completely stopped washing and brushing my hair," followed by why I dove into the ocean, and then John worked for hours to detangle my hair—"and here I am today."

Kyle listened and validated. The half-spoken message from Kyle was that everything I thought I did right was all wrong. After locking the salon door, he stood behind me hour after hour, vertical, never showing signs of back or leg cramps, pulling through the possession that represents physical health and vitality to women. The sun went down and the moon came up. Using his fingers to detangle and pull knots out of my hair, he worked his way up by starting with the ends and then going to the roots. We heard a knock at the locked door. It was John. He surprised us and brought me dinner. The three of us talked casually like old friends telling fun stories on a holiday trip. But my stomach twisted in grief, not wanting to acknowledge the fact I was going to completely lose my hair.

John told me months later how Kyle concealed the damage. Standing on one leg, trying to be inconspicuous and extending the other leg in a whip-like fashion, he would brush his foot along the floor to kick away all the ripped-out hair droppings. Kyle acknowledged the desperate situation I was in by applying this constructive coping technique that took remarkable balance and quick reflexes to make sure I wasn't seeing my headful of hair falling underneath our feet.

If I had met with any other stylist, I would have been told: "I'm sorry, there's nothing we can do for you. We will need to cut this mess off and then you'll have to get used to a short haircut, and that won't last long either." Kyle was giving me time to process the situation and circumstance, to understand and cope with my loss. It was all therapy: the detangling, telling stories and talking to me. It was a buildup. It had nothing to do with earning money, as he barely charged me anything. It had everything to do with Kyle giving me his time as I was coming to grips with reality.

At 9:30 p.m., when I looked straight ahead in the mirror, I discovered that no matter how hard I tried or how much I cared, there would be no "good ending." I had made decisions without having perfect knowledge. The situation was imperfect and I would need to make a quick decision. Kyle then leaned over me and sweetly said, "What do you think, are you ready to get your hair cut?" He was willing to sit with me in silence for a minute. This man could have told me five hours before: "Look, I'm sorry. There's nothing we can do. You obviously will need to cut your hair off." Kyle had intentionally chosen a life different from his family, who worked on auto factory lines in Grand Rapids. Yet, here he stood on his feet for five tedious hours of labor to gently show me that the path of least resistance would be the best option.

The short haircut lasted only a few weeks. By December 2, I was down to only two patches of hair around my ears. A few days later, I had only a few strands left on my head. I got in touch with a woman who made soft purl-knit, cashmere beanie hats with faux fur pom-poms. These are what I wore day and night for the next several months.

Still, there was something deeper than just my hair loss, and less definable, that frightened me. I had entered the fight that would test the logic of my life. It became a private lesson in how much power I *perceived* I had and my inability to manifest things by an act of will. I am pretty sure I willed myself to stop growing at the age of 12. I found a way to leave home at age 14 without running away, willed my great-grandmother to live to 104 so she would meet my first-born son, and willfully found a home on one of the nicest streets in Nashville. This time, there would be no triumph, just disappointment. The plan would be diverted. I would not be keeping my hair by an act of will, nor my eyelashes and eyebrows, which fell out six weeks *after* my final chemo treatment.

My approach to my hair was a step-by-step plan of action, proving adaptable at each step, just like an escalated, exaggerated physical improv comedy exercise: something that had started out simple got complicated and tangled up, like the conveyor belt scene in *I Love Lucy*. I wasn't ready to give up control, accept what was happening and concede to this breast cancer.

There was a piece that would help me decrease stress and avoid unwanted emotional suffering—a wig. The wig would give me a gentle reprieve; people would smile at me for what felt like the right reasons. Other people's worry, pity and expressions can sometimes make us feel out of control. Looking normal after my hair loss would give me mental strength, as though I was not being pushed around or reacting to the transient occurrence of other people's strong feelings. I didn't want anyone's visible worry to take away from my focus on the day-to-day details of breast cancer surgeries, chemo, my business and my body's ability to heal. Creating a "normal outside" made me calmer and gave me more energy.

And for practical reasons, I *needed* this wig for business meetings with clients.

So off I went to the luxury wig market. I bought a killer wig—as realistic as possible. A hand-tied, fully silk-based lace wig that was branded as "100 percent virgin Eastern European hair," with an open-lace front to create a genuinely natural front hairline. (The term *virgin*, I later learned, refers to the human hair not having been subjected to processing.) It was made from *real* human hair—woven in the same direction as natural hair growth, and it would need washing and styling. Kyle would color it. What I purchased would not be mistaken for a wig.

And then, in the midst of my quiet grief and suffering, I'd experience a brief moment of fantastical wonder with Andrew styling my wig. It would be like watching van Gogh use oils, that special

159

point of view given to me as if I was the canvas—personally experiencing his work and seeing his expressions as he created. If I could go back in time, I'd strap a camera to my head and capture footage of Andrew as he styled the front hairline of my wig.

As part of embracing my wig, I was instructed to work out in it so that it would start to move with me. So wearing my wig, I boxed with Sena, jumped rope, lifted weights with Royce, and took classes at Pure Barre.

Round Eleven

SEEN AND UNSEEN

Sena had been out of town once again to train at Floyd's gym, or what he called "camp," and had just returned to Nashville for his big fight. On a Saturday morning, the unimaginable happened. There are certainties I had told myself: *the best fighters notice everything, they have an astute awareness and keen eye for detail, like superheroes.* But time passes, and looks change. We mean different things to different people. After a year of seeing my face up close on Mondays, Wednesdays and Fridays—working with mitts, hitting the bags, seeing my worried look or my needing a nod of approval, how I raised my eyebrows or tightened my cheekbones when I was supposed to keep a neutral gaze, how I might have rolled my eyes when I was exhausted, expressions that showed confidence or showed I was ready—on that Saturday morning in late November, Sena no longer recognized me.

It had only been two months or so since I last saw him. Not being recognized hit at my deepest desire to be seen. His inability to see that it was me shut down my own perception of myself being special and standing out. Now I understood: I was seen as average or possibly just adequate. Without my hair, I realized I wasn't a familiar face to him, which stunned me. He literally didn't know who I was. Even when looking right at me, staring and studying my form for a few minutes as he walked around the track at the Y, telling himself, *She looks like she knows what she is doing, impressive form.* He couldn't see his own work—my form and technique that he was partially responsible for. The odyssey I had gone through had totally changed me.

Sena not recognizing me at the Y was a stark reminder of how different I must have appeared to others without being aware of it. It was the first time I had gone out of the house without my wig. I had temporary bionic, perfectly formed, bubble-like boobs and no hair left on my head, but my scalp was covered up with my purled, sparkly gray beanie. I had to reintroduce myself to him. I walked over to the track and greeted him with a big hug. I had to remind myself that I was not the person I was when we first started to train.

For Sena, there was no need for acknowledgment, external validation or recognition from even one of the greatest boxers of his generation. For others to see him and his own worth was simply expected. The legendary former five-division world champion Floyd Mayweather had been matter-of-fact, not afraid to see and point out greatness. He just strolled straight up to a younger Sena, making eye contact and saying, "I like your stuff." These four words were powerful coming from Mayweather. Sena wasn't bragging, just shrugging and sharing it with me in a pragmatic way while wrapping my hands: Floyd had noticed the obvious, Sena's greatness, which was already apparent to the rest of the world.

When Sena wrapped my hands in the mornings and tied the laces around my boxing gloves, it felt like the beginning and closing of parentheses. With a focus on protecting my wrists and hands, we really saw each other, talked to better understand each other about our thoughts, feelings, beliefs, and motivations. One morning, I asked him what it was like to train at the Mayweather gym: did he ever run into Floyd? My imagination took over, seeing his life in Las Vegas—a setting sun, a boxer's thrilling, glittery world. Impervious to anything flashy, Sena could have been describing Floyd's gym like any old strip mall gym in rural North Dakota or Oklahoma—he wasn't bedazzled by anything. The details he shared were dull words that implied it was just another work place with concrete floors and after work, he cooked traditional Ghanaian meals of "beans, plantains and chicken" for his Puerto Rican trainer Rafael Ramos (who wanted Sena to marry his sister). Sena might have been a kid from the countryside seeing Las Vegas as just all wrong, sad and sick, a place that needed to be sanitized. I got the picture that the grueling workouts at Floyd's gym kept his world insulated and mundane.

Then he shared a simple story that stuck with me forever and, in my mind, seemed incredible (at least to a woman who was blind to authority at the time). With no cars in sight and simply walking across the steet in Las Vegas, Sena saw two white police officers rushing toward him to arrest him for jaywalking. What pardoned him, I learned, was that he sounded like the Queen. They were smitten with his distinct and stylish Ghanaian English accent, a different pronunciation from all the West African countries, and they were happy to let him go. I began to wonder about any other African-American man, whose outcome might be unfortunate because of how he pronounced his A's or used stronger R's.

Not being recognized by someone with whom I'd had so much interaction was new for me. It led me to recall my misplaced feelings of what it was like to not be seen, as I sometimes felt less loved and appreciated by John, the faithful husband and a man who could have authored the book, "Confessions of the Best Father." Never did I think John had his own problems. The irony was I'd later learn that there was no one more important to him than me.

I had struggled for his attention, trying to break through what I mistakenly saw to be his indifference at times. His singular focus in walking in the front door after work was on the order of the home, anticipation of what might be out of place, or what potentially was going to get dropped on the floor at dinner. There were times I had been feeling denied in my marriage, dismissed. I had slowly shut down. I woke up some mornings and imagined my family without me. If I were out of the picture, John and his new wife, a lawyer or doctor, would be laughing together, proudly writing checks for private school tuitions, beaming together on luxurious family vacations, and no longer worrying with the pesky, falling-apart needs of our 1924 home. All I can say now is whatever his negatives, he certainly rose to the occasion and gave his all to me just when I needed it desperately.

John and I had met for the first time in a suburban mall bookstore on a Thursday night. He'd left the cash register, led me to the back of the store as if I were a suddenly-arrived VIP guest, and took the requested book off the shelf. His face showed no judgment about my selection of the book—about seeking a higher level of self-understanding—and he gently placed it into the palms of my hands. Like a gravitational game, we kept running into each other around town, our eyes locking. We would have puppy love moments. He'd give me a lift to college classes on the handlebars of his red Bianchi bike. He showed his dedication by waiting for me outside my classroom doors. When he took off for France to study again there for a year, there'd be miles between us, but they didn't mean a thing. In calligraphy, he'd write close to a hundred letters professing his love, telling me he "felt connected to me" in our long-distance relationship. We spent a month together wandering the streets of Paris—in the mornings filing down a circular staircase behind Parisian drag queens, all of us guests at the Hotel Tholoze for $17 a night. And then at night, we climbed the steep hill leading up to the hotel by the windmill in Montmartre, at a time when the neighborhood felt more like a village.

On our wedding day, we were surrounded by thoroughbred horse pastures and said our vows inside a 1782 stone church with ties to Mary Todd Lincoln's grandfather. Here people would witness my biggest example of hesitation, all based on my own loss of control and management over an event that had been tightly scripted, while getting ready to say the magical words to the love of my life, not knowing whether I was going to be able say my vows or whether I would flee. The minute the preacher spoke, I sensed trouble. The wedding ceremony lines I crafted to be spoken and heard by all, reflected my identity and values and were an important part of making what was to be the most perfect day of my life. It now all felt reckless, an injustice deeper than anything I had expected to feel on my wedding day. Rather than hearing "Oohs" and "Aahs" from the congregation I heard laughter. I knew I was making the best decision of my life marrying John, but I started crying at the altar while a possibly drunk preacher stumbled through the first sentence of my orderly script, "We gather here today to join this man and HIS woman ...," and then hearing the congregation howl. I stood there. Nothing seemed funny at all. The squeeze of John's hands and the eye contact he would make, as if saying *We've come this far, you can do this*, would stay with me for the rest of my life. His steady look of confidence reframed the situation. These same eyes and gesture showed up when babies were born, when I wanted to fire difficult clients but our family needed the money, and as we navigated life's hardships.

I felt this same connection with him when I got hit with the hardest punch of all: breast cancer. That's when I started seeing that my husband's perfect love had been there this whole time. How he consistently and quietly took on all the chores I hated, brought me coffee in bed, filled our gallon jugs with fresh distilled water every week, took care of our cars, could find anything lost, pumped water out of our basement, fixed our washer or dryer, and helped our sons with math. Now John was in a lockstep march with me, the fighter. A man intent on duty, with an innate sense of calm and perspective, never deviating from his love for me. John had helped me clear out my old ways of eating over the weekend when I began my macrobiotic diet. He bought and labeled containers for our pantry like a professional organizer and stocked them with all my new foods and grains. This man understood the complexity, preparation, and time involved in cooking my meals. He selflessly, for the next eight months, did all the grocery shopping and quietly cleaned up behind me, washing my pots, pans, dishes, knives, and cutting boards, and saved vegetable remains for broth.

For two people who had been on separate paths, we started to do just about everything together. It was the most perfect decision of my life, marrying John. It took cancer and about 30 years to see this.

Round Twelve

SUCKER PUNCH

After chemo infusion number 11, my new oncologist gave me the ultimate gift: her decision to end it all. I was spellbound for a moment, ecstatic. I wanted to run out of the patient room, spread my arms, and skip. I felt that this appalling journey was done and I had been awarded a unanimous decision. The decisive call was based on the worsening of my neuropathy—a pin-pricking and burning of the nerves in my fingertips and toes that lit fire right into my bones, as though someone was forcefully holding my fingers in a candle's flame and my toes in scalding hot water.

Joyful, I thought to myself that this would be my last experience with all the equipment around, above, on top of, and in me—the IV, glass tubes, sterile line and port. There'd be no more chemo drip from tubes going into my bloodstream, every cell in my body exposed to the yew tree-inspired poisons, fluids from a plastic bag entering my body, the accumulation weakening my immune system. No more half-days of sitting in a recliner with a heated white cotton blanket on my lap, taking away my life. I saw a clear path, seeing that I was the designated favorite, expecting the win. In my mind, with this new decision, I had won the fight. I thought I had been successful in my planning and now I saw progress. In each round, I was doing exactly what Sena had told me to do: "Execute with confidence" or "Remember every punch I throw is intended to set up the next one."

Now all I would need to focus on was my recovery from 11 rounds of chemo, and then I would have my breast reconstruction surgery in six weeks. I had been training hard as a bald woman—my head sporting a soft, lightweight, slouchy gray cashmere hat covered in tiny fake pearls and glints of sparkles. Or on days I wanted to feel like a normal woman, I'd wear my wig and baseball cap. Three days a week I jumped rope, jogged a mile on a treadmill with five-pound weights in my hands, alternating between jabs and crosses, in addition to rounds of hitting the mitts with Sena. On the other three days, with a band looped around my feet, I followed Royce's instructions: start off with his foundational quad exercise—RDLs—then onto deadlifts, shoulder shrugs, bent-over rows, squat presses, curls, upright rows and chest presses. All of my training felt miraculous at the time.

I was down to the final round. Only one more surgery to go.

But there was a surprise in store for me and more confusion up ahead. Bad guys, of course, don't make a coherent threat. This new situation made me question what was real and what was not. I was given a warning. Something dreadful was arriving, there would be a vile, proud, dark opponent. Christy had warned me about those fighters who fight dirty and don't play by the rules. I was eating clean, staying physically and mentally strong and choosing the right corner. This new opponent would be the deceptive tricky fighter, brutally mauling opponents, perhaps the kind of fighter caught wearing hand wraps stiffened with plaster or other illegal paraphernalia.

I knew things were not right with this new invisible presence. My internal ticking was off when the sun would set. I fell into bed, cold. I moaned. My teeth chattered, I shook uncontrollably, and experienced being chilled to death, deep into my bones, my flesh ice-cold, but somehow also drenched in sweat with a high fever. There was a separation of my body and soul. This started to become the norm. I'd become so weak, finding myself on my hands and knees, crawling around on the old hardwood kitchen floor, thinking about the new me with a cardboard identification tag attached to my big toe. My pale skin was cold to the touch. Dampness and rain made it worse. A fiery chill penetrated deep into my bones. My mind was murky.

The body part that became a key player in the spiritual history of humanity, according to the Bible, was sending me an explicit warning that no one in healthcare could accurately read. It started with a flat, red rash that looked like pinpricks, covering my right rib area. I was in turmoil, not wanting to be a bother to anyone, but I forced myself to seek help. The doctors and nurses reached a quick conclusion: "an allergic reaction to laundry detergent." And they sent me home. The nonchalant diagnosis left me in self-doubt, wondering if my mind might be playing tricks on me, or if I was thinking straight. I was desperate to believe the worst was over. But deep down, there was no confusion in my mind that something vile was causing a deterioration.

At the end of January and early February, I started sending notes to Sena and Royce to cancel my training, saying: *I have had some weird things happen this week with my health. I got an infection*

171

with flu-like symptoms on Wednesday—it's still hanging on today, maybe had a terrible allergic reaction to the meds—my entire chest and abs area looks like I've been burned red.

One day I'd be running on the treadmill, and the next day sending a note: *Hi Sena! I hope your day has been a good one. I am very sick, not sure if flu or what—have not felt like this in a very long time. I am sorry but will need to cancel tomorrow's session with you and pick back up next week. Thanks for your understanding.*

Phone conversations with Royce would be about my perseverance and his encouragement to be strong. He'd ponder: "Wait a minute, let me understand this. You are lying in the bed now because of a little rash? And after all your training during chemo?"

I became terrified to tell anyone about how I was feeling. I started quietly slipping into a place of feeling alone, floating somewhere between life and death, my soul loosening, as if each blow of breath would be my final one. When I prayed and meditated in the mornings, I sometimes felt the breath of a bearded Jesus in front of me and a hand on my head. Other times, comforting me, there was a presence of my younger self. I no longer saw the flaws in my house that hadn't been painted in 14 years, but only the energy of my kids and husband as they moved from room to room. It wasn't sadness or depression; it just seemed like life was drawing to a close.

What I didn't know was that there was a Strep B infection in my port. At night, somewhere between dreaming and a waking life,

I was now smothered by a new urgency: the stubborn force of my maternal great-grandmother telling me I was entering into a place outside of time. It was her presence that had comforted me when I was suffering in my darkest moment during chemo, chasing away the evil beast of the night that was stealing away my life by sweeping her willful hands over my body. Now, drifting off to sleep, I was jolted as she came to me with an urgency to take action. She was predictable, reawakening me every night like an intruder. Her presence said there had been a lot of wasted time and hesitations in my life.

I would take a trip to Kentucky, without knowing I was about to die.

She was obstinate, stern, pestering me to get going and quit finding excuses to not learn more about a missing man in her life, a father who had left with no memories to give her son. Her new nightly visits told me I was indeed transitioning to the afterlife. She was warning me that things were coming to a close and I had to go back and read all those letters. I had told myself that if I ever got out of chemo, I would track down all the details of my maternal great-grandmother's story and the missing man in her life. Now I felt compelled to fulfill one filial duty, to resolve her story before letting go.

The one event I felt haunted by and needed to understand was the full story of the disappearance of my great-grandfather C.M., who left a wide hole in our old Kentucky family, with his absence reverberating for generations. There were generations of white lies, half-truths, rumors about him "being a good man," misinformation and falsehoods that no one seemed to forget or get straight.

For years, the letters to her and about her always had rested in the back of my mind, at times residing as an obsession or creating a feeling of emptiness. After she died, I rescued the protected letters from meeting a blazing fate, as they were about to be flung into the farm's burning trash heap. They had been safeguarded for almost 90 years, each one neatly stored in its individual envelope in a large, flimsy box. She was the central figure in a rich story. Only my great-grandfather C.M.'s letters survived. There were plenty of witnesses and all the details were caught on stationery and postcards. Years after I sat in her lap, the dead continued an existence in me.

Long ago, we'd had a face-to-face in her tiny white kitchen. I asked what seemed to be a simple question, causing her to tear up and shake her head. She side-stepped my question, saying it was just too hard for her to talk about it. I walked away both shocked and ashamed that I could make a 90-something-year-old woman feel trauma from so long ago.

We shared the same name—Kelly—and we both had a large collection of French love letters from our husbands. I had my collection from John. She had hers from C.M. Mine had a happy ending. For her, there was no joyous reunion. Things could never go back to the way they were before. With her new nighttime visitation ritual, her letters felt more relevant. I started to become consumed with questions about things left undone and unre-solved for her that would have to be dealt with. I started to feel better and confident about making the drive to Kentucky for a personal mission to read the letters.

***

For several days, each morning at 10 a.m., I climbed a marble spiral staircase at the Kentucky History Center and then walked through a monitored research room to look for reserved carts with my name on them. I had arranged for the donation of our family letters to this entity years ago. Sitting all day in a state archival institution, wearing my beanie, I opened his envelopes and read his letters, now stored in acid-free archival boxes, neatly processed in files with plastic paperclips. Reading what were once *my* letters, I'd be supervised by two librarians and allowed to sit with only one box at a time.

The elegant penmanship was deceiving, making you feel certain about his character—a proper, honorable gentleman—because of the perfect mathematical proportion of his graceful slant, upstrokes and spacing of his handwriting. He signed "CM Perkins" at the bottom of each letter, multiple pages of folded red and blue ink on stationary that read, *American YMCA, ON ACTIVE SERVICE, with the American Expeditionary Force.* They were slipped into envelopes first addressed to Chicago, then later to Kentucky. It's hard not to be enamored. At first, he composed tender and loving letters, not wanting to be apart from her. You see evidence that builds your belief that he is principled—he even wrote letters and postcards to her sisters and brothers and mother.

They began in September 1918 with sweet expressions of love, when he'd refer to her as "girlie." There's nothing about combat, the course of the war. You understand there is the heartbeat of an unborn baby. He says he'll be coming home any day now. You read between the lines that she can't sleep and "has the blues." There'd be more assurances that he'll depart at the end of the month—every month. She gives birth to their baby boy away from her family's Kentucky home. You feel her frailty. He says to her, "How I would like to be with you … I hope the baby is fat … with lots of hair and big eyes. I certainly will be glad for the day of our departure."

There was a filled-out new mother's baby book recording the baby's firsts and seeing the growth of the baby boy. He was born weighing eight pounds, three-fourths of an ounce, and in six months, would weigh 23 pounds. There was a list of messages of congratulations, gifts, and a written recording of the baby's first outing. C.M. says he is making every effort now to get back home. But he's too shifty. You know she's no fool. The war ended long ago and still he stays, even walks in Versailles on Sundays. She fears he's been untrue.

Requests asking her to borrow money for business interests become a theme for him. You see the stark difference in their realities—he travels around Europe, but she is now a single mother, unwanted and no longer welcomed in his parents' home.

Intentions change. He's cowardly. The letters now are written on Parisian hotel stationery. I feel her simple desperation. Repeatedly she'd be asked to sail over one day, he'd be making big plans for her and the baby. Then he would become aloof. His possible infidelity weighed heavy on her heart. There'd be government documentation around his disappearance, seemingly just off having a great adventure. She was bitter for a good reason.

I now wanted to spit on his grave, I hated myself for being led on, forever believing him, being so naïve, gullible and over-trusting. In the end, there'd be no joyous reunion. A cablegram saying *CM died at midnight March 26, 1925 in Glen Ellyn Illinois* was sent to her beauty salon on the second floor of the Lafayette Hotel.

I didn't make it through all the letters before I drove back to Nashville, reaching a new understanding. I felt I had accomplished my mission. Even though I couldn't change the outcome, I had gotten to the bottom of the truth.

After the trip, all my energy was put toward my California client and the COO's planned trip to Nashville for a rare face-to-face planning session. A month earlier, I had been brilliant in pulling off my part—a *me being perfectly normal* meeting over wine in a darkened restaurant bar booth, wearing one of my sparkly cashmere beanies fitted tightly on my blown-out wig. She spent hours telling me about her breakup with her boyfriend after their trip to Bali. I dropped her off at her hotel and felt like I had nailed it, even negotiating a renewed big contract.

Here she was, unfortunately for me, back in Nashville again. I had been meticulous in my preparation for our upcoming meeting.

Yet, I felt wobbly as I took my wig to get it blown out and styled at 8 a.m. My pale face and insides decimated by the poisons, I wanted to wrap myself around this marketed European virgin-harvested hair to feel a sense of normal. My hair looked great, but my face showed that chemo had taken its toll. I struggled with washing the wig in the bathroom sink that morning. I made the bad decision to put the wet wig on my head wrapped in a white towel, and drive in the cold just up the road to get it blown out. My wig—made of thick, full hair—resembled a 20-year-old's, styled as if I was going to a ball. But wearing the cold wet wig for too long had caused me to start shaking. Walking through the glass door entrance of the mall for some makeup touch-ups, I was on overload as I tried to manage how best to step onto the escalator. I was overwhelmed looking at the white, shiny tile floors, kiosks, and people sipping coffee walking toward me with shopping bags.

An hour later, wearing my wig with a smile and energetic voice, I was visibly sinking in front of the company's COO. After the meeting, I held on to railings and walls to get to the car. Once inside, I shook uncontrollably in the parking garage. Nothing made sense to me. I felt devastated by how I had showed up in the meeting after going to such lengths to look physically normal. I knew I had blown it with my client. This was the client who had previously voiced concern about *what if something happens to you?* I was barely able to drive the straight one-mile route back to my home. My thinking was off. I didn't want to be a burden to John or anyone else by calling for help. I kept thinking the worst was over, I was no longer in chemo treatments, and I should be okay now.

Sitting in my driveway for an hour, I was weak, depleted and shaking. Getting out of the car just didn't seem like an option. I eyeballed the front door, encouraged myself with self-talk that getting inside would be a straightforward process, that I could do it. I reduced things to the basics: turn off the car, get out, stand up, shut the car door and walk the 20 feet to the front porch. *What could be simpler?* I questioned. I forced myself to swing my legs out of the car. Staggering and counting out loud to a repeated rhythm of five, I managed the two sets of steps up to the porch, feeling as though it was an incredible, miraculous achievement.

Once inside, I lay down, feeling my life was surely coming to an end. It felt like I had taken a devastating right hook to the body, my opponent swatting me down with a left hook to the head, sending me stumbling back into the ropes. I was wobbly, disoriented and wincing. I experienced punishing symptoms of what it might feel like the day after a tough fight, feeling 100 years old with hurt muscles, my head bursting, and a damaged rib. Surely, I'd get right back up after hours of rest, feeling no damage.

Days after this disastrous client meeting, I woke up feeling surprisingly good and trained with Sena the day before my final breast reconstruction surgery, long scheduled for February 8. This surgery would be stage two of the reconstruction process, the last step. For the past several months, I had walked around with inflatable boobs with a bionic structure, shape and size. These were tissue expanders, temporary, anti-gravity, what felt like concrete boobs. Initially they were deflated silicone implants inserted immediately after my double mastectomy. Once a week I had watched these temporary boobs get inflated and expand. My tissue expanders had done their job—stretching my breast skin, tissue and muscle. Both boobs were now at the desired reconstruction size.

The night before my final surgery, I experienced a cruel situation. There was no sleep before the big day. I had a temperature of 103, chills, and night sweats. Helplessly, I moaned and had an outbreak of the shakes in bed as if possessed by something scary. I knew things were not right but saw no other choice than to go to my scheduled surgery. Somehow John would gather me up, and we would find ourselves at the hospital at 5 a.m., sitting together in the lobby.

I was delirious and silently upset about how undignified I looked with pale skin, physically ravaged, sporting patches of discolored redness. I was overly anxious and obsessed with one thought: *my death is imminent and I was unsure how all this was going to play out.* My body chilled again. I sat quietly and uncomfortably as people who knew why they were there stared at me as if they were doing research. I heard John say "No" to me when I mumbled, asking him if I could please rest my head in his lap.

My name was called and I staggered forward. Things were different this time. This was the same place as before, but this time it felt distorted: the same pre-operative area with doctors and nurses in green scrubs, the taking away of my clothes in a plastic bag, the open-to-the-front hospital gown, standard questions, compression devices with an attached air pump squeezed onto my legs, my young handsome plastic surgeon briskly passing my area carrying the same elegant Prada briefcase as before, mapping out the surgery by pulling out his handy Sharpie to draw patterns on my breasts and stomach. What was different was my casual attitude that I just no longer cared and that no one in the hospital understood what was happening. I struggled with the haste and suddenness of feeling that this was the end of my life.

I spent time chatting with my kind anesthesiologist about Alex's ACT preparation. He shared vivid details of his son's experiences serving in the Israeli Defense Force (IDF), and we made the connection that his son had been in the same graduating class as my older son, Will, at Montgomery Bell Academy (MBA). It was hard for me to fathom, a young man the same age as Will, recently a part of our world, forgoing the traditional route of college and now part of the Israeli-Palestinian conflict. I killed time before my surgery scrolling through my boxing and strength training videos and photos.

I saw my lawyer-preacher friend Robin dash into a high-security pre-operative area minutes before, as she did for each of my surgeries, with the same gravitas and singular focus in what had become a ritual. I could have been in a locker room where the coach had just entered with a pre-game speech. She would respectfully instruct whoever was getting ready to be a part of the operating theatre—whether it be surgeons, anesthesiologists, an infectious disease team, nurses or medical students—to all hold hands in a circle and say a prayer, appealing to a higher spiritual being for help during my surgery. Despite the myriad of variables—different hospitals, doctors, time of day, type of procedure—it was always predictable. She would call me the night before each surgery to find out the time, place and all the details, and then miraculously show up minutes before. She would take a breath and have the undivided attention of the room. She created a sense of urgency to make them understand what they were "playing for," bringing focus by reminding them of their purpose. No one questioned her authority and were all agreeable to participate in this prayer just for me.

There was a sudden reversal of course, minutes before surgery. Calmly, sweetly standing over me, my plastic surgeon raised a red flag, sharing the news that there would be no surgery today. My white blood cell count was elevated from its usual three to 17. My body was fighting an infection. I felt so ashamed. I was such a burden, a bother to my surgeon that I had wasted his morning, his valuable time. Guilt-stricken, I asked him if he'd ever had this happen. When he responded no, I felt worse about myself and walked out of the hospital with my head down.

Because of John's insistence and planning, there were cultures and blood tests taken by my oncologist after leaving the hospital. Curled up in a ball on my side on a patient table, motionless, I transformed the patient room into a calm, pitch-black emptiness with John sitting in a chair. While waiting, I could have slipped into the night's expansive darkness of the desert consumed with nothingness, total blackness. I could breathe now with an absence of light, feeling as though I was becoming invisible. I had no thoughts but wrestled with one notion: *Was it true?* Was I laying on a table at 5 am this morning being prepped for my final surgery? I took a short, dreamless nap. An abrupt bright light from the corridor blinded me, a reminder of where I was. I was in a lit room and in pain. I opened each eyelid separately, working to adjust to the intensity of the lights being turned on, my pupils dilating. Adam, a nurse at my oncologist's office, moved me around quietly, calmly examining me, as though I was a large immobilized animal stunned by a tranquilizer gun.

I was sent back home where I slept for 15 hours straight, from 3 p.m. to 6 a.m. I awoke feeling a deep pause, renewed in what seemed to be a picture-perfect home and new mental freedom. I felt as though I had made it out alive, off a high mountainous cliff that was dangerous to scale. I was okay but faced a new zig-zag path with the derailment of my reconstruction surgery. I was now catapulted into a space of not knowing what was happening.

Two hours later, I got a call from Adam explaining that I would need to come to the university hospital for more blood tests. *It was a Saturday, I thought, on the weekend. Really? Couldn't I get a break from all the health stuff and all the needles?* After more discussion with Adam, I complied. Confident, I told John I had this, got myself dressed, drove my car a mile or so down the road, parked it in a garage and felt proud that I could find

183

the makeshift entrance area to the infectious disease team. With each heavy step, I presumed there'd be routine bloodwork, a quick turnaround, then back home again for lunch.

Once I entered the infectious disease area, the unthinkable happened. I was sat down in a patient room and was told I would need to be admitted into the hospital because of a Strep B infection in my port.

The fear of going to a doctor's office or a cancer infusion center had stayed with me, but what seemed even more treacherous was the idea of entering a hospital as a patient—for an unknown extended period of time, cut off from the wider world, subject to elaborate controls, confined to a bed or room, the regular two-hour check-ins by kind but tired overworked nurses. My inner self was so fragile that I hated how my normal proud self might be processed through the apparatus of the healthcare structure, being reduced, stripped of my dignity and breaking my sense of self.

The media interviews I had landed related to evolving hospital threats and patient safety ran through my head. I had helped script *They don't know what they don't know...* scenarios that might make unwanted news headlines for hospitals. I had coached clients on how best to communicate the most serious dangers around patient risks in hospital patient care. I had heard first-hand about all the noise in a hospital administration that created confusion. I was responsible for writing corporate messaging to position my healthcare and technology company clients to offer peace of mind to hospitals. And now I found myself on the other unbearably personal side as a patient.

One of my earliest childhood memories formed my unease with university hospitals, triggered by being hit with the distinctive, harsh odor of disinfectant and being smuggled in at the age of four. In 1971, hospitals had a customary rule: Children were banned from visiting patients. The fatal scale of our tragedy would bend that rule: My sister and I were treated as exceptions. We ended up in a white boxed patient room in a university hospital where we visited our 8-year-old big brother, Sid. We saw the aftermath: our active brother trapped in a full white plaster body cast with his broken right leg elevated in a sling. In the press, Sid would be the eight-year-old who fell to Earth, the only survivor to tell the story of a plane's vertical dive onto a runway from directly above people's heads. He was the survivor of the plane crash that killed our father. Physically, my brother would recover completely from the crash, cared for by our great-grandmother, but my dread of hospitals remained.

So off I went, four decades later, to being a patient in another university hospital. While my world felt convoluted, I tried to hold on to a sense of normalcy in all my communications to family and a few friends. John sent concise messages to family and a corner of friends: *We got the cultures from yesterday's visit— appears to be strep b infection in port—they want to administer antibiotics through IV and monitor her for 24-48 hrs—she is near our house.* At the time, it was hard for me to grasp the seriousness of my situation—even with a Rocephin IV drip, used for life-threatening infections, administered in my arm—nor was I told by the doctors.

When I was admitted to the hospital this time for the infection in my port, there were things I was determined to hold onto, like my power and my sense of being, to stare down this new challenge. I'd be compliant while keeping my self-autonomy mixed with denial. My ways of comforting myself involved keeping my sense of self through the continuation of my work, eating clean, and fitness. My plan was to take these things with me. But I found myself inside an institution where I would give up basics like food, water, and information.

I was not allowed to eat or drink until dinnertime each day in anticipation of an unscheduled surgery to have the infected port removed. My only desire in the hospital was water. My tongue was so dry and heavy throughout each day. Every second, I wanted to scream for water. I felt I no longer had saliva. I tried with every thought to curb my hunger. One day, when I was just about to eat dinner, I got the call and was wheeled down for surgery—the removal of my infected port.

Even while starving in the hospital, I somehow continued to run my PR business from my room, not saying a thing to my clients—coordinating conference calls, continuing to land media stories and building out a new PR strategy. My decision to not disclose what was happening to me was a simple financial calculation—I did not want to lose business. One morning, I walked down the hall to the nurse's station and made an unusual request of the Head Nurse—I wanted to reserve an executive conference room. I needed this conference room so that I could confidently present my new PR strategy to a healthcare client's CEO, CFO and COO. John would hold down the fort in my hospital room in case a doctor showed up looking for me. I ended the teleconference presentation by asking if anyone had any questions, getting only feedback from the leadership team of how impressed they were with my strategy.

Some days while waiting for the removal of the port, I'd run the hospital's flights of stairs with an IV in my arm to keep fit. I struggled to get information. Had the doctor ordered the removal of the port? How high or low was my white blood cell count? How many more days would I be deprived of food and water, and how many days had it been already?

The many blood draws in little glass tubes made me feel as though I was dealing with an empty gas tank, sputtering in the middle of nowhere, late at night. Nurses were no longer looking at the veins in my arm for drawing blood, but called for backup. They'd resort as a last option to the fingers on my left hand. (For the rest of my life, I could only have blood drawn from my left arm, the one not at risk of lymphedema. Lymph nodes had been removed from the right arm, rendering it off limits.)

Around 10 p.m. one night, I sent one of my text messages to Sarah in Massachusetts, who checked in with me just about every day. She sensed my despair when I ended the message with, *I wish you were here!! Sending lots of love to you.* A few minutes later, she had a flight booked to Nashville from Boston and spent the next afternoon with me in my hospital room, sitting beside my bed. I warned her ahead of time that she might not recognize me.

The impersonal—and what felt like smug—crowd of residents dressed in white coats conferenced around my bed each morning with a different attending physician. While everyone else was standing except me, I attempted to ask questions of an emotionally detached physician, while different representatives of the student assembly tried to impress one another with their medical knowledge. What I longed for was a doctor to sit down and talk with me. The communications with physicians reminded me of our 22-hour flight to Thailand in 2003, where the captain made two dramatic announcements at once with constant shifts in decision-making: that our plane was running low on fuel and that we were flying through a tsunami. One minute he'd say we would reroute and fly to Korea, and an hour later, he would turn the plane around and head to Sapporo, Japan, and then land in Nagasaki.

The patient room environment included beeping monitors, hourly check-ins, forced awakenings, blinding lights, opening of the door. Staying by myself at night, I longed to go home. As much as I hated John seeing my chest wounds from surgeries, it was more painful having him see me in a hospital bed. He would bring a late lunch each day after getting a go-ahead that I could eat and then return with Alex after school for dinner. Unable to go home with them, confined to a bed, I had thoughts of escaping. One night my anguish reached a new level when Alex visited my room and shared that he had not made his school's baseball team. I told John I would have rather been whipped with a stick than to see Alex's face sharing his news.

I lived through the hospital stay of five days, and then ten days of John administering an IV for me at home. It all took its toll on me. A few weeks later, I no longer resembled my old self—a graying of eyebrows, no eyelashes, no hair, the blotchy red patches that resembled an old Siberian woman. My eyes looked like the eyes of someone who has been to other side—one foot on Earth, one foot on the other side of death. All of this seemed to be another woman's life. I saw the head of the university hospital's infectious disease team a few weeks later and she casually said, "Do you remember toxic shock syndrome from the '80s? That is what you had."

It was a mystery as to where and how I got the infection. I let it go and never asked any perplexing questions of anyone. My gut told me my body needed serious time to recover and I put off the anticipated final breast reconstruction surgery for late March. I felt desperate due to the amount of alone time in my home, not leaving for days, but I continued to run my business. I sent a note to Sena saying: *Started feeling a little discouraged this past week. It's been a little rocky after my blood was contaminated... but I have been stable over the past few weeks. My reconstruction surgery is scheduled for this Friday.*

And then on the last Friday of March, I'd lie on a patient table in the same mid-town hospital's pre-op room, listen to Lizzo, and type a text to Sarah minutes before going to the operating room: *I'm all marked up! My surgeon just came in and found some fat in the back part of my legs for boobs!!*

After what I thought was to be my last surgery, I could no longer cover up and fake normal. I slowly embraced the phrase: *Beauty is found in the unraveling of things.* My neighbors and more people around me were startled by seeing this new me, my face ravaged from the infection, all the antibiotics, chemo treatments and with less than an inch of mostly graying hair. I dropped wearing the wig—never to see it again. I lost that one client's contract renewal in May. I decided to take a sabbatical from my work and heal.

It wouldn't be the final surgery. I was surprised a few months later to find out there would be one more surgery needed in December, 2019. My new boobs needed more fat. This whole ordeal had started the summer of 2018. But in the last procedure, I felt like a heavy hitter who landed a knock-out punch.

In early May, I came back to my training with simple stretches at Royce's gym. By mid-month I was resuming my strength training with Royce twice a week with soft duck feather-like, wavy, spikey-in-front hair, listening intently as he frequently said, "Good job" and "Improving 1% daily." His words were important. But visualization was an effective practice for Royce. He used visual cues, knowing how they stick in a person's long-term memory, to motivate, reach a deeper understanding and leave a longer impression. He wanted me to grasp my new strength and how my body had healed from trauma and how I was getting closer to where I wanted to be in life. Six months after my final chemo and twelve weeks after my reconstructive surgery, he started sharing videos of my pullup shrugs and explosive pushups—so I could see the lumbar muscles in my back and triceps. He wanted me to know how my balance had been restored by looking at my own Bulgarian split squats, a lunge forward on one foot with the back foot elevated on a plyo box.

I'd go four months without boxing. I wouldn't resume training with Sena until the end of May. My first few days back, my facial expressions showed I was concentrating so hard, but still cautious of any impact. I clearly recalled the 40-punch combo, but I was gently tapping, barely hitting his mitts. By October, I started to see how I was punching with new power, was crisper than ever before with my movements, sharper in my swivel angles and pivots, speedier, and I could consecutively master what was once a 40-punch combo that became the 82-punch combo. I rarely needed to stop and think, as I seemed more clear-headed, with an increased confidence and effective reactions.

I was getting ready to do that one weightlessness thing, that one euphoric rush—something causing time to move slower and my whole universe to come into a better focus. As I got into a boxing stance, I had a particular view as well. Standing face-to-face with a super middleweight fighter who looked superhuman, I paused to reflect on his personal mantra he held onto strongly: *It's only a matter of time, I'm already there.* I then led with a double jab, slips to the right and left, hooks, triggers, upper cuts, body shots, swivel angle to the left, rock backs, cross, pivot, hooks, crosses, and double rolls, ending with a double right jab.

I looked up and breathed deeply, realizing I just had done something I wasn't capable of doing before. I smiled and let that thought *I'm already there* sink in.

Round Thirteen

POST FIGHT CONFERENCE

It's been over a year since my last surgery and two years since I finished chemo. My hair has grown back to its original length but in spiral curls that I never had before. I'm still strength training with Royce and practicing Jeet Kune Do with Richard. I've taken up dance again after 30 years, and also weight lifting because of Alex.

I have stepped away from my PR business and have embraced my new self: never again Just Kelly. Now I am Sarah's friend, Will and Alex's mom—not the same, because I am now better able to appreciate the young men who loved me fiercely through all eleven rounds with their individual supportive selves. I'm Kelly, the woman honored to be cherished and protected through the battles of breast cancer by my husband John, who loves me more intentionally (with all my many scars, too).

I am a survivor, one whose arms were held overhead by all of these and countless others; one who knows I can tackle the worst and still rise victorious, waiting for the victory bell inside the boxing ring of my journey.

After being hit so hard, I had to pick myself back up and avoid the dreaded 10 count. I needed healing, I needed to get back in the ring and show life that I was not done, not knocked out in the final round like so many before me.

Cancer is a formidable adversary. You never really win against cancer. You hope for a draw, to fight another time, to train and battle and be ready, if you have to return to the ring again. You are ready.

Boxing has taught me discipline, greater awareness and an approach to life that requires a commitment to process and demands mental, physical and spiritual fitness. It is grueling and exhausting, but it ultimately prepares you for the fight for your life.

Appendix A:

SEASONAL HEALING FOODS

SPRING

Liver/Gallbladder:
barley, leafy greens, traditional umeboshi plums

SUMMER

Heart/Small Intestines:
bitter greens, salad

LATE SUMMER

Spleen, Pancreas/Stomach:
millet, sweet squash, round vegetables

AUTUMN

Lungs/Large Intestines:
brown rice, hardy greens, pungent roots

WINTER

Kidney/Bladder:
adzuki beans, miso, hardy roots

Appendix B

HERE IS WHAT I ATE:

Sea Vegetables
Nori
Wakame in soup
Kombu cooked in beans and vegetable dishes
Arame
Dulse
Agar-Agar in desserts

Flour Products
Udon, somen noodles
Black bean noodles
Shirataki

Grains
Brown rice
Groats
Quinoa

Grain Variations
Quinoa, brown rice, groats

Condiments
Mitoku traditional Umeboshi plums—ate often, half a plum a
day, either straight or steeped in hot water

Pickled Food
Sauerkraut and kimchi

Beverages
Kukicha twig tea after each meal

Green tea

Spring water between meals

Alphay antioxidant mushroom coffee

Dandelion tea

Aloe vera juice

I was to avoid vegetable juices, alcohol, sparkling mineral waters, carbonated water, cold drinks, sugared or stimulant beverages

Oil
Sesame oil

Olive oil

Coconut oil

Avoid canola oil

Regular Every Day
Barley miso 3 years old, light and dark

Whole clove of garlic

Unrefined white sea salt

Umeboshi paste, plums, vinegar

Brown rice vinegar

Ginger, cinnamon, turmeric

Lemon

Herbs

Sauerkraut and kimchi

Nuts
Almonds

Walnuts

(Supposed to soak my nuts and seeds for anywhere from 20 minutes to three hours for increased digestibility)

Seeds
Pumpkin seeds

Sunflower seeds

Chia seeds

Flax seeds

Hemp hearts seeds (raw)

Animal protein
Orange roughy

Cod

Flounder

Haddock

Ground Fruit (between meals)
Berries

Watermelon

Tree fruit
Granny Smith apples

Supposed to soak my nuts and seeds for anywhere from 20 minutes to three hours for increased digestibility.

Sauerkraut and kimchi

BREAKFAST:

Miso soup:

I used barley and other types of miso

I made vegetable miso soup just about daily with a small amount of wakame with shitake mushroom with leafy greens, daikon and carrots, adzuki beans, garnished with scallions.

Groats

Adzuki beans

Snacks

Mochi

Hummus

Acknowledgments and Thanks

I could not have written this book without my corner:

Laura Anne Turner, Sena Agbeko, Royce Fentress, Richard Goodloe, Christy Halbert, Ph.D., Robin Kimbrough Hayes, Sarah Rulnick, Kyle Brougham, Andrew Pentecost, Dr. Mei Zhao, Virginia Harper, Susan Waggener, Judy Wachs, Sobeida Salomon, Mary Helen Clarke, Molly Secours, Melissa Grove, Beth Tallent, Andrew Maraniss, Tom Nielsen, Ph.D., Michelle Prentice, Jennie Fields, Max Warren, Xander Williams, Natalie Watterson, Annette McNamara, Chris Amato, Michael Catalano, Sid Motley, Rong Yan Guan, Leemon Williams, Debbie Howard, Jocelyn Limmer, Traci and Joe Gallivan, Gene Reese, Horace Fentress, Adam Stater, Dr. Karl VanDevender, Dr. Jean Ballinger, Dr. Jacob Unger, Dr. Vandana G. Abramson, Dr. Regina Offodile, Erin Drury, Mandi Kowal, and Randy Harris

I'd like to acknowledge the influence of these books:

The Fight, Norman Mailer
On Boxing, Joyce Carol Oats

9 780578 246154